THYROID HEALING

Learn how this gland regulates our body's mechanisms, prevents dysfunction, and heals it with natural remedies and proper nutrition

BY

GLORIA ROBERTSON

Copyright © 2020 by Gloria Robertson

All rights reserved

This book or parts thereof may not be reproduced in any form, stored in any retrieval system, or transmitted in any form by any means—electronic, mechanical, photocopy, recording, or otherwise—without prior written permission of the publisher, except as provided by United States of America copyright law.

Table Of Contents

Thyroid Healing Diet Plan 1
1. Thyroid Gland And Its Functions 1
   1.1 Introduction 1
   1.2 Structure Of The Thyroid Gland 2
   1.3 Functions Of Thyroid Gland 3
   1.4 Hormones Produced By Thyroid Gland 3
   1.5 The Regulator Of Thyroid Gland; The Master Gland 4
   1.6 The Relationship Of Furnace And Thermostat, Pituitary And Thyroid Gland 6
   1.7 How The Thyroid Gland Works? 7
   1.8 The Biochemistry Behind Thyroid Hormone 7

2. Thyroid Malfunctions: Hyperthyroidism And Hypothyroidism 10
   2.1 Types Of Thyroid Malfunctions 10
     2.1.1 Hyperthyroidism 10
     2.1.2 Hypothyroidism 10
     2.1.3 Goiter 11

2.2 Why Thyroid Hormone Levels Are Crucial? 12

2.3 Symptoms Of Hyperthyroidism And Hypothyroidism.. 12

3. Causes Of Thyroid Abnormalities 16

3.1 Causes Of Hypothyroidism..................................... 16

4. Genetics Of Thyroid Diseases 29

5. Lifestyle, Diet And Nutrition For Thyroid Abnormalities 31

5.1 Foods That Are Bad For Thyroid Function 37

5.2 Complete Diet Plan For Managing Hypothyroidism... 40

5.3 Complete Diet Plan For Managing Hyperthyroidism 41

5.4 Lifestyle Changes For Hypothyroidism 46

6. Thyroid Medications, Do's And Don'ts 49

7. Genetic And Environmental Basis Of Thyroid Dysfunction 51

7.1 Genetics And Thyroid Disorder 52

7.2 Common Genetic Variation 52

7.3 Genetics Of Thyroid Function 54

7.4 Variation In Thyroid Genes And Their Clinical Manifestations 55

8. Nutrigenomics And Thyroid Disease 57

9. Oxidative Stress And Thyroid Dysfunction 62

9.1 Effects Of Oxidative Stress On Thyroid Gland ... 64

9.2 The Best Antioxidant Diet For Controlling Thyroid Dysfunctions 66

10. Problems Related To Thyroid Diseases And Their Treatment Via Diet... 70

10.1 Thyroid Disorder And Depression 70

10.1.1 Thyroid Hormone Metabolism In The Brain.. 71

10.1.2 Thyroid Dysfunction And Related Neuropsychiatric Disorders 72

10.1.3 Thyroid Hormone Status In Patients With Depression.. 73

10.1.4 Thyroid Hormone Supplementation In Depression.. 74

10.1.5 Treating Thyroid-Related Depression With Diet.. 75

10.2.1 Treatment For Thyroid-Related Fatigue.......... 78

10.3 Thyroid Dysfunction And Sleep Disorder.......... 79

10.4 Thyroid Dysfunction And Anemia...................... 79

10.5 Thyroid Dysfunction And Iron Deficiency 80

10.6 Lifestyle Changes For Coping With Problems Related To Thyroid Dysfunction 80

11. Thyroid Dysfunction And Pregnancy 84

    11.1 Hyperthyroidism In Pregnancy 84

    11.1.1 Effect Of Hyperthyroidism On Mother And Baby 86

    11.1.2 Diagnosis And Treatment Of Hyperthyroidism In Pregnancy 86

    11.2 Hypothyroidism In Pregnancy 87

    11.2.1 Effect Of Hypothyroidism On Mother And Baby 87

    11.2.2 Diagnosis Of Hypothyroidism During Pregnancy 87

    11.2.3 Treatment Of Hypothyroidism During Pregnancy 88

    11.3 Postpartum Thyroiditis 88

    11.4 Diet For Coping With Pregnancy-Related Thyroid Dysfunction 89

12. Thyroid Disfunction And Hair Loss 92

    12.1 Relationship Between Thyroid And Hair 92

    12.2 Symptoms Of Thyroid-Related Hair Loss 93

    12.3 Treatment 94

    12.4 Natural Treatments And Home Remedies 94

13. Thyroid Dysfunction And Weight 97

    13.1 The Link Between Hyperthyroidism And Weight Loss 98

13.2 Relationship Between Hypothyroidism And Weight Gain 99

14. Other Thyroid-Related Dysfunctions 101

14.1 Goiter 101

14.1.1 Various Causes Of Goiter 102

Iodine Deficiency 102

Autoimmune Disease 102

Less Common Causes 103

14.1.2 Diagnosis Of Goiter 104

14.1.3 Goiter Surgery 106

14.1.4 Best Diet For Goiter 106

14.2 Thyroid Nodules 107

14.2.1 Symptoms Of Nodules 108

14.2.2 Causes Of Nodules Formation 108

14.2.3 Diet And Lifestyle Changes To Reduce Nodules 111

15. Role Of Microbiota In Thyroid Diseases 115

15.1 Link Between Thyroid Hormones And Microbiota 116

15.2 Gut Microbiome And Thyroid Disorder 118

15.3 Role Of The Gut Microbiota In Autoimmune Thyroid Diseases 119

15.4 Role Of Microbiota In Therapy Of Thyroid Disorders 123

15.5 Role Of The Gut Microbiota In Metabolism Of Thyroid Hormone.. 124

15.6 Healing The Gut To Improve Thyroid Function 127

15.6.1 Increased Intake Of Fermentable Fiber.......... 128

15.6.2 Use Of Probiotics 128

15.6.3 Keeping A Check On Sibo Or Other Gut Pathogens... 129

15.6.4 Practice Gut-Friendly Regime 129

16. Hashimoto's Protocol And Diet Plan For Thyroid 131

16.1 Thyroid Diet Plan.. 131

16.2 Three Pillars Of Diet Plan....................................... 132

16.2.1 Pillar 1: Remove What Is Damaging And Toxic For A Thyroid 133

Pillar 2: Add Food To Boost The Immune System, Detox And Improving Thyroid 136

16.2.3 Pillar 3: Create A Balance In Eating And Lifestyle 138

16.3 Recommended Meal Plan For Hypothyroid Individual... 139

16.4 Things To Consider Before Adopting Any Diet Plan 142

17. Treatment Of Thyroid Via Detox 143

17.1 Detox With Caution 152

17.2 The Risk Associated With Detoxification With Hypothyroidism.. 153

17.3 Thyroid-Friendly Ways To Boost Detoxification 154

18. Treatment For Thyroid Dysfunctions................ 157

18.1 Best Treatment Options For Hypothyroidism . 157

18.1.1 Hormones Replacement Treatment 158

18.1.2 Medication With Synthetic T3 And T4 Hormones Combination.. 159

18.2 The Best Treatment For Hyperthyroidism........ 160

18.2.1 Beta-Blockers... 160

18.2.2 Surgery (Thyroidectomy) 161

18.2.3 Radioactive Iodine 161

18.2.4 Anti-Thyroid Medications 162

References.. 164

Thyroid Healing Diet Plan

1-Thyroid Gland and Its Functions

1.1 Introduction

The thyroid gland is one of the most vital glands in our body and medically it is known as the glandula thyreoidea. It is considered the essential hormone gland as it plays a central role in the development, metabolism, and growth of the human body. It functions to regulate various functions of the body by continuously releasing a specific number of thyroid hormones into the blood.

The amount of thyroid produced by the gland is dependent on the energy needs of the body. That is why when the body needs more energy as in case of growth, cold and pregnancy, the gland produces a higher amount of hormone to meet the metabolic needs of the body.

1.2 Structure of The Thyroid Gland

The thyroid gland is present in the neck region, at the front, just under the voice box (pharynx) which is sometimes known as Adam's Apple (Figure 1). It has a butterfly-like shape with two side lobes. These lobes are present against and around the windpipe (trachea) and are connected at the front by a special tissue known as the isthmus. However, in some individuals the isthmus is absent and there are two separate lobes of the thyroid. On average, the weight of the thyroid is between 20 and 60 grams and is around 2 inches long.

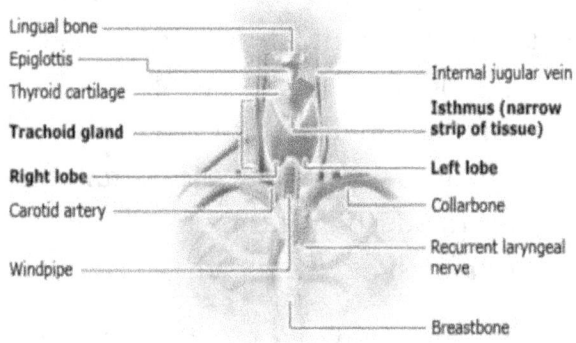

Figure 1. The location of the thyroid gland in the body

The thyroid gland has two fibrous capsules on its sides (Figure 2). The outer capsule is attached to the muscles of the voice box and various nerves and vessels. A loose connective tissue is present between the inner and the outer capsule, which allows the movement of during swallowing.

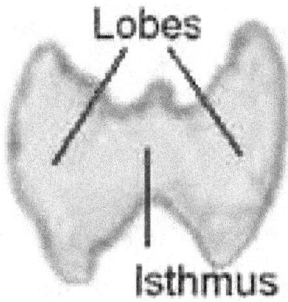

Figure 2. The simplified structure of thyroid gland

The thyroid tissue is comprised of tiny individual lobules enclosed in layers of connective tissue. Many small vesicles (sacs) called follicles are present in these lobules. These follicles store thyroid hormones in the form of small droplets and release them when needed by the body.

1.3 Functions of Thyroid Gland

The primary function of the thyroid gland is to control metabolism. It plays a diverse role in the body and some of the vital body functions that are regulated by thyroid hormone include heart rate, body weight, breathing, nervous system, body temperature, menstrual cycle, muscle strength, and cholesterol levels.

1.4 Hormones Produced by Thyroid Gland

There are three distinct hormones produced by

the thyroid gland. These include

- Triiodothyronine, known as T3
- Tetraiodothyronine, also known as thyroxine or T4
- Calcitonin

Physiologically only T3 and T4 are pure thyroid hormones. They are synthesized in the follicular epithelial cells of the thyroid gland. The main building block of T3 and T4 hormones is iodine that we get through our diet. Iodine is an essential trace element as it is not produced by the body and is absorbed into the blood from the food in the intestine. And is carried to the thyroid gland. Calcitonin is the third hormone produced by the thyroid gland. It is synthesized by the C-cells and is involved in bone metabolism and the regulation of calcium levels in the body.

1.5 The regulator of Thyroid Gland; the Master Gland

The requirements of the thyroid hormone in our body vary considerably. Sometimes it needs more thyroid while at others it needs it in a very minute amount. So, who tells the thyroid gland to make more or less hormone? The master gland, pituitary gland (a small peanut-sized gland present under the brain) and the hypothalamus in the brain are responsible for the synthesis of the required amount of thyroid hormone.

The hypothalamus releasing TSH Releasing Hormone (TRH)sends signals to the pituitary gland to order the thyroid gland to produce more or less T3 and T4 by either increasing or decreasing the production of a hormone called thyroid-stimulating hormone (TSH). Moreover, there is a certain amount of thyroid hormone present in the blood that is attached to an inhibitory protein. And T3 and T4 are released from the protein when the body needs more amount of hormone.

The pituitary gland regulates the thyroid gland in the following two ways (Figure 3):

- When the blood T3 and T4 levels decrease the pituitary gland produces more TSH and mediates the thyroid gland to release a higher number of thyroid hormones.
- When the blood T3 and T4 levels are high, the pituitary gland releases less TSH to the thyroid gland to decrease the production of these hormones.

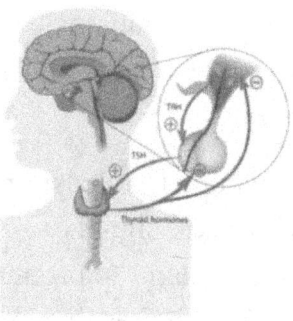

Figure 3. The regulation of thyroid gland by the pituitary gland

1.6 The relationship of Furnace and Thermostat, Pituitary and Thyroid Gland

As discussed, the thyroid gland is under the regulation of the pituitary gland (the master gland). When the level of T3 & T4, becomes too low, the pituitary gland releases the Thyroid Stimulating Hormone (TSH). This hormone stimulates the thyroid gland to produce an increased amount of hormones. TSH mediates the thyroid to manufacture and secrete T3 and T4 and leads to a rise in blood levels.

The increased level of thyroid hormones in the blood is sensed by the pituitary gland and responds by a decrease in the production of TSH. This relationship between the pituitary gland and thyroid gland can be considered similar to furnace and thermostat, where the pituitary gland acts as the thermostat and the thyroid gland is the furnace.

The thyroid hormones, T3 and T4 are like heat. When the level of hormones increases, the heat gets back to the thermostat, and the thermostat is turned off. As the level of thyroid hormone decreases, the body cools, and the thermostat is turned back on with an increase in TSH and the furnace produces more thyroid hormone which equivalent to more heat. The pituitary gland is controlled by the hypothalamus with produces TSH Releasing Hormone (TRH) which tells the pituitary gland to send a signal to the thyroid gland and release TSH.

1.7 How the Thyroid Gland Works?

The thyroid gland is part of an elaborate endocrine system, which consists of various glands that synthesize, store, and release hormones into the bloodstream so the hormones can reach the cells of the body. The iodine from the food is used to make T3 and T4 hormones. It is very crucial that the levels of T3 and T4 are neither too high nor too low. The hypothalamus and the pituitary glands in the brain communicate to maintain a balance of T3 and T4 in the body. And allow the optimum functioning of the thyroid gland.

1.8 The Biochemistry behind Thyroid Hormone

The primary function of the thyroid gland is quite simple: to process the iodine that is found in our diet and transform it into thyroid hormones: thyroxine (T4) and triiodothyronine (T3). In humans, the cells of the thyroid gland are the only cells that can absorb iodine. Once inside the thyroid, iodine is attached to the amino acid tyrosine to make T3 and T4.

T3 and T4 are then released from the thyroid into the blood and are transported to various parts and organs of the body where they primarily regulate the energy-related metabolic processes that involve the conversion of oxygen and calories to energy. Thyroid hormones are considered central to the metabolism of the body as every cell in the body is dependent upon thyroid hormones for the regulation of their metabolism. The two hormones are produced in different ratios by the thyroid gland, as a normal thyroid produces about 20 % T3 and 80% T4. The hormonal strength of the two hormones is also different as T3 is about four times stronger thanas T4.

The T3 and T4 hormones function to rise the basal rate of metabolism. They make cells of the body work harder and consequently; they need more energy. This has the following effects on the body:

- A rise in body temperature.
- Faster pulse and stronger heartbeat
- Food is used up more quickly because of the

release of energy stored in the liver and muscles
- Maturation of the brain in children
- Improvement of Growth in children).
- Activates the nervous system that boosts the senses and leads to better reflexes and improved concentration.

2-Thyroid Malfunctions: Hyperthyroidism and Hypothyroidism

2.1 Types of Thyroid Malfunctions

Despite being a highly regulated gland, thyroid functions can sometimes be dysregulated. This dysregulation of the thyroid gland leads to increased or decreased production of thyroid hormones. There are two conditions that are related to an abnormally functioning thyroid gland, they are known as:

- Hyperthyroidism
- Hypothyroidism

2.1.1 Hyperthyroidism

An overactive thyroid is when the thyroid gland makes more hormone than needed by the body. This condition is known as hyperthyroidism.

2.1.2 Hypothyroidism

An underactive thyroid is when the gland is

unable to produce sufficient hormone that is required by the body. This condition is known as hypothyroidism.

2.1.3 Goiter

The malfunctioning of the thyroid gland is not limited to increased or decreased production of the thyroid hormone. Sometime the gland itself may swell and become larger in size and may cause abnormalities in the individual. This thyroid gland abnormality is termed as goitre and it can be of two types,

- The enlargement of the whole thyroid gland, known as diffuse goitre
- The formation of time lumps, known as nodules on the gland, known as nodular goitre

The nodular goitre can lead to increased or decreased production of thyroid hormone. If the nodules produce an increased number of hormones, then such nodules are termed as "hot" nodules. While, if the nodules are producing less amount of hormone as compared to normal levels than such nodules are known as "cold" nodules.

Mostly, the enlarged thyroid or the presence of nodules are non-life-threatening conditions and are only rarely tumorous.

2.2 Why Thyroid Hormone levels are Crucial?

Till this point, we have learnt that the levels of T3 and T4 in the blood are highly regulated. But it is now important to understand they the mere presence of these hormones is not sufficient, but their levels are very essential. As we know that when T3 and T4 reach the various cells of the body, they regulate the metabolic rate in that tissue or organ. The physiological effects of T3 and T4 are to regulate the heart rate and how quickly the intestines process food.

So, if the levels of T3 and T4 are low, the heart beats at a slower than normal rate, and one can have constipation and weight gain. But if T3 and T4 levels are high, the heart beats at a rapid rate and can lead to diarrhoea and weight loss. These and other physiological effects of the level of thyroid hormones in the body make it very important that we keep a close check on our thyroid levels and monitor the related changes in our body. Further, a special examination, the thyroid scintigraphy, is done to check the presence of nodules and their effects on the production of thyroid hormones.

2.3 Symptoms of Hyperthyroidism and Hypothyroidism

The hormonal imbalance leads to various

complications that are manifested in the body in the form of various physiological symptoms. However, every individual would have any number of these symptoms and have varying degrees of severity of these symptoms. The combination of symptoms that may appear in an individual and their respective severity depends on two factors:

- The extent of increase or decrease in the hormone levels
- The time period for which the body has been exposed to the hormonal imbalance

Symptoms of Hyperthyroidism

When the body produces too much thyroid hormone, it can suffer from the following symptoms and conditions.

- The person can develop anxiety which is accompanied by mood swings, irritability, and short temper.
- It can lead to increased heart rate (palpitations), nervousness, breathlessness, fear and hyperactivity.
- It can lead to increased sweating or and can develop extreme sensitivity to heat and high temperatures.
- It can affect the placement of eyes and can

cause protrusion (bulging out) of one or both eyeballs.
- It can lead to disorientation, shaking and trembling in hands.
- It can also cause cosmetic damage which primarily includes dried and brittle hair accompanied by hair loss.
- In women, it can alter the menstrual cycle and can lead to light menstrual periods or can stop them causing missed periods.

Symptoms of Hypothyroidism

When the body produces too less thyroid hormone, it can suffer from the following symptoms and condition:

- The person suffers from general weakness, fatigue, and tiredness.
- It causes sleep disorders and the person fails to get a good night's sleep.
- It leads to sudden and unexplained weight loss. And in already obese individuals, it causes difficulty in losing weight.
- It causes the skin to appear dry, pale and rough.
- The person becomes oversensitive to cold and is not able to tolerate low temperatures.

- It leads to muscle weakness and causes subsequent muscle aches and muscle cramps. It can also cause pain in joints.
- It leads to mental disorders, such as depression, crankiness, feeling gloomy and unwanted.
- It can lead to digestive disorders such as abdominal discomfort, loss of appetite and constipation.
- It causes brain fog and the person have difficulty concentrating and memory loss.
- In women, it leads to frequent heavy menstrual periods, which lead to considerable blood loss. This can result in anaemia if left untreated.

3-Causes of Thyroid Abnormalities

3.1 Causes of Hypothyroidism

The lack of the required amount of thyroid hormone can negatively affect the metabolism of the body. There can various underlying causes of hypothyroidism. Some of the most widely studied factors that can lead to hypothyroidism are:

- Autoimmune disorder
- Treatment of hyperthyroidism
- Thyroid surgery
- Radiation Therapy
- Use of certain medications

In the next section, we will briefly discuss the causes of hypothyroidism.

❖ Autoimmune disease

One of the most common causes or factors that leads to hypothyroidism is an autoimmune disorder termed as Hashimoto's thyroiditis. An autoimmune disorder is defined as a disorder of the immune system when the immune system of the body produces antibodies that attack own tissues. Sometimes these antibodies are produced against the tissues of the thyroid gland, which leads to death and destruction of the cells of the gland This loss of thyroid cells leads to a decrease in the production of thyroid hormone.

Hashimoto's disease is a multifactorial disease and various researches have suggested that it results due to genetic and environmental factors. Other risk factors of Hashimoto's disease are discussed below:

1). Age

Age is considered a risk factor for developing this autoimmune disorder, as Hashimoto's disease is more prevalent in middle-aged individuals.

2). Sex

Hashimoto's disease has been known to affect women more frequently as compared to men.

3). Exposure to Radiations

Exposure to various environmental radiations increases the risk of developing Hashimoto's disease.

4). Other Autoimmune Diseases

The presence of other autoimmune diseases such as lupus, type 1 diabetes or rheumatoid arthritis increases the risk of developing Hashimoto's disease.

❖ Side effects of hyperthyroidism treatment

Individuals with hyperthyroidism are mostly treated by giving radioactive iodine and other anti-thyroid medications in order to reduce the unwanted levels of thyroid in the body. And to get the function of thyroid back to normal. But in some cases, this treatment does not go as planned and leads to a much lower thyroid hormone production as compared to the normal levels. This condition becomes permanent and leads to hypothyroidism.

❖ Thyroid surgery

Surgical removal of all or a large part of the thyroid gland can reduce or stop hormone production. Such individuals suffer from hypothyroidism to no thyroid hormone and have to take thyroid hormone for the rest of their lives.

❖ Radiation therapy

Radiation therapy to treat various cancers of the neck and head region can negatively affect the functioning of the thyroid gland which can lead to reduced thyroid hormone production.

❖ Medications

Certain medications, such as lithium that is used to treat behavioural disorders can affect the thyroid gland and lead to hypothyroidism.

❖ Congenital disease

In some cases, the babies are born with a faulty thyroid gland or the thyroid is completely absent. In most cases, this defect in the development of the thyroid gland occurs due to unknown reasons, but some babies carry a defective gene for thyroid disorder.

❖ Pituitary disorder

This factor is quite rare and involves the failure of the pituitary gland to make a sufficient amount of thyroid-stimulating hormone (TSH). In most cases, this occurs due to the presence of a benign pituitary gland tumour, which reduced its ability to produce TSH.

❖ Pregnancy

In some cases, pregnant women may develop hypothyroidism during or after pregnancy, known as postpartum hypothyroidism. This occurs due to the production of antibodies against their thyroid tissues. If this condition is left undiagnosed and untreated, hypothyroidism can lead to an increased risk of premature delivery or miscarriage. Sometimes, this condition can also lead to preeclampsia, which is characterized by aa significant rise in the blood pressure of pregnant women, which can adversely affect the health of the fetus.

❖ **Iodine deficiency**

As thyroid uses iodine for the production of T3 and T4 hormones. The deficiency of iodine in the diet can drastically decrease the ability of the thyroid gland to produce hormones. Iodine is present naturally in seafood and in plants grown in iodine-rich soil and is now added to table salt, which has significantly eliminated the issue of iodine deficiency, especially in the USA.

3.2 Risk Factors of Hypothyroidism

Hypothyroidism can be developed by anyone and at any age but there are certain factors that are considered as risk factors for thyroid reduced function. And individuals who have any or multiple of these factors are at increased risk of developing hypothyroidism. They are discussed below:

- Hypothyroidism is more prevalent in women

as compared to men, so women are at more risk of developing this disease.
- Individuals who are older than 60 years are considered to be at higher risk.
- Individuals who have a family history of thyroid disease are considered to be at increased risk.
- Individuals with an autoimmune disease, such as lupus, celiac disease or type 1 diabetes are at an increased risk of developing hypothyroidism.
- Individuals who have been given radioactive iodine or thyroid-repressing medications are at an increased risk of developing the disease.
- Individuals who have been exposed to radiation at the neck or upper chest area are included in the high-risk group.
- Pregnant women or who have delivered a baby in recent months can develop the disease.

3.3 Complications of Hypothyroidism

In some cases, the patients of hypothyroidism can suffer from a severe life-threatening condition. This happens in those cases when the symptoms of hypothyroidism go undetected and the disease progressive without any check and treatment. In hypothyroidism, when the body is required to make a specific amount of thyroid hormone and the pituitary gland make a large amount of thyroid-stimulating hormone (TSH). This extra signal of work creates a load on the thyroid gland and the high amount of TSH cause the gland to become enlarged. This leads to the formation of goitre, known as compensatory goitre. If this condition is left untreated, it leads to severe hypothyroidism and can lead to life-threatening heart failure, depression or coma.

Some other complications of hypothyroidism are discussed below:

❖ **Mental health Problems**

One of the earliest signs of untreated hypothyroidism is depression as low levels of thyroid take a toll on brain health. The individual may also suffer from poor cognitive abilities and slow brain functioning.

❖ **Peripheral neuropathy**

Long-term unaddressed hypothyroidism can lead to severe damage of the peripheral nerves, which is known as neuropathy. In normal individuals, the nerves carry information from the brain and spinal cord to the rest of your body. Peripheral neuropathy leads to pain, restlessness and numbness and in the different areas, especially in arms and legs.

❖ Myxedema

Myxedema is a life-threatening condition, but it is quite rare. It occurs in individuals who have been suffering from chronic hypothyroidism and leads to the development of severe cold intolerance and lethargy which can lead to profound drowsiness and unconsciousness.

❖ Infertility

Thyroidal hormonal imbalance affects the ovulation process in women. This may lead to infertility issue if hypothyroidism remains treated.

❖ Birth defects

Women with hypothyroidism are more prone to give birth to babies with various complications and defects as compared to healthy mothers. Such babies are at risk of developing cognitive, developmental and various metabolic abnormalities. Babies born with thyroid abnormalities have a good chance of recovery with early diagnosis and proper treatment.

3.4 Causes of Hyperthyroidism

Hyperthyroidism is caused by various factors and

it can manifest itself in varying severities depending on the number of underlying causes and conditions. Some of the most common causes of hyperthyroidism are given below:

- Graves' Disease
- Thyroiditis (inflammation of the thyroid gland)
- Abnormal secretion of TSH
- Functioning adenoma and toxic multinodular goitre (TMNG)
- Excessive iodine intake
- Excessive intake of thyroid hormones

❖ Graves' disease

The most common cause of hyperthyroidism is Graves' disease. This disease is characterized by the presence of an overactive thyroid gland that produces more than the required amount of thyroid hormone. Graves's disease is caused as a result of the loss of the ability of thyroid gland to respond to the control of pituitary gland through the TSH. Graves' disease is hereditary in nature and can be transferred from affected parents to children. Moreover, women are more likely to be affected by the disease and Grave's disease has been known to affect women five times more than men.

Graves' disease is an autoimmune disease. The immune system start to produce antibodies against various regulatory molecules of the thyroid glands, for instance, antibodies against thyroid-stimulating hormone known as thyroid-stimulating immunoglobulin (TSI antibodies), TSH receptor antibodies and thyroid peroxidase antibodies (TPO) are released into the blood that leads to alteration in thyroid function.

❖ **Symptoms of Graves' disease**

Graves' disease has the same symptoms as hyperthyroidism, along with the presence of skin lesions and eye diseases. Eye diseases (ophthalmopathy) can occur after, before, or at along with the hyperthyroidism.

❖ **Triggers of Graves' disease**

There are various triggers for the Graves' disease. These include:

- Exposure to radiations in the neck area
- Smoking
- Stress
- Medication
- Infection with bacteria or viruses

A standard, nuclear medicine thyroid scan can be

used to detect Graves' disease. And the presence of increased uptake of radioactive iodine shows abnormalities of the thyroid gland and indicate Graves' disease. Moreover, a simple blood test can be used to detect elevated levels of TSI.

❖ Thyroiditis (inflammation of thyroid gland)

The second most common cause of hyperthyroidism is the presence of inflammation in the thyroid gland. It may occur due to viral illness, a condition termed as subacute thyroiditis. This condition is marked by the presence of symptoms like fever and sore throat, accompanied by pain in the swallowing process. The thyroid gland becomes tender to touch. And the person becomes subjected to generalized pain in neck and shoulders.

Further, a condition called lymphocytic thyroiditis may also occur, which is characterized by the accumulation of white blood cells (WBCs) in the thyroid gland. In both cases, the inflammation makes the thyroid gland "leaky," and an increased amount of thyroid hormone enters the blood. Lymphocytic thyroiditis commonly affects pregnant women and may appear after delivery in around 8% of cases. The hyperthyroidism can last from 4 to 12 weeks of the postpartum period and is sometimes followed by a phase of hypothyroid that may last for several months. However, most of the affected women heal to normal thyroid function after within a year.

- ❖ **Function.ing adenoma and toxic multinodular goitre**

The formation of lumps and nodules can occur in the thyroid gland, and this process can be accelerated with age. In most cases, these lumps don't produce thyroid hormones and hence are considered harmless and benign. But in some cases, the nodule can become "autonomous," that means that the nodule develops the ability to produce thyroid hormone independently is not under the control of pituitary gland.

The probability of a nodule to become autonomous is increased significantly if its size is greater than 3 cm. The presence of a single independent nodule that is producing thyroid hormones, it is termed as functioning nodule. If the number of such functioning nodules is more than this condition is called a toxic, multinodular goitre. The presence of functioning nodules can be detected with the help of a thyroid scan.

- ❖ **Excessive iodine intake**

Iodine is used by the thyroid gland to make thyroid hormones. But in excess, iodine can lead to hyperthyroidism. Hyperthyroidism caused by the overdose of iodine is most prevalent in patients who already suffer from an underlying thyroid disorder. The use of certain medications, including amiodarone that is used to treat heart problems, contain high levels of iodine and is found to be linked with thyroid function defects.

❖ Abnormal secretion of TSH

A presence of a tumour in the pituitary gland may lead to the production of atypically high production of TSH (the thyroid-stimulating hormone). This results in unnecessary signalling to the thyroid gland to release thyroid hormones. This condition is quite rare and can be linked with other pituitary gland dysfunctions. Various tests can be performed to assess the release of TSH from the pituitary gland and detect the presence of altered secretion of TSH.

❖ Excessive intake of thyroid hormones

The intake of too much thyroid hormone is quite common and is one of the common causes of hyperthyroidism. This can be accidental and mostly goes unnoticed by the doctors or patients. However, some people abuse the drug in order to achieve other goals, for example, weight loss.

4-GENETICS OF THYROID DISEASES

Genetics is as an important factor for the determination of thyroid hormone concentrations in the body. Moreover, it has been found that various genes have been identified in humans which have been linked with increased susceptibility to autoimmune thyroid disease. Heritability studies involving thyroid diseases show that around 67% of circulating concentration of thyroid hormone and TSH concentrations are determined genetically. This suggests that there is a definitive genetic basis that forms a set or standard point for the intra-individual variation in the levels of thyroid hormone.

Various genes have been found that are determinants of thyroid levels in the body, these include genes for F-actin-capping protein subunit beta, phosphodiesterase 8B, iodothyronine deiodinase 1 and the TSH receptor gene. However, these genes have little control of the variability of thyroid hormone in the body that suggests that there are other epigenetic factors and mechanisms that can control the function of the thyroid gland.

Some genes, including iodothyronine deiodinase 2 and the TSH receptor, that influence the thyroid function also have a wide range of roles in the body. For instance, they are involved in the control of developmental phenotypes, regulation of bone health, neurological development and longevity. These findings show that the complex nature of thyroid hormone and its diverse functions in the body. The hereditary nature of autoimmune thyroid disease that runs in families and the identification of such genes is considered to be vital to allow prognosis and detection of thyroid disease in members of the affected family.

5- Lifestyle, Diet and Nutrition for Thyroid Abnormalities

The concept of using diet as medicine is gaining interest all over the world. Nutritionists are using the healing powers of dietary nutrients to control and treat various diseases. The fact that the thyroid gland is dependent largely on a dietary component, iodine, makes thyroid disorders one of the most widely studied disease by nutritionists. It has been found that many nutritional factors and food components play a significant role in the optimizing the functions of the thyroid gland. Nutrient deficiency and excess, both, have been linked with triggering and progression of thyroid diseases. One can significantly improve his thyroid functions by following a certain diet with the recommendation of a nutrition expert and physician.

Moreover, the lifestyle which includes daily routine, eating habits, sleeping routine and physical activity have been found to play an important role in developing thyroid dysfunctions. It has been proposed that by adopting a healthy lifestyle, that includes good diet and exercise, one can protect the body from this hormonal disorder and can also decrease the symptoms of any kind of thyroid dysfunction. Lifestyle changes can help in managing and reducing the damaging effects of hyper or hypothyroid on the body.

Some of the highly recommended food components and lifestyle changes that act as strong regulators of the thyroid gland are given listed below:

- Iodine
- Selenium
- Vitamin B12
- Vitamin D
- Goitrogens
- Exercise

In the next section, we will discuss some of the most vital nutrients and food components that have been proved to have regulatory effects on the functions of the thyroid gland.

Iodine

Iodine is an essential nutrient in the body and has a significant role in thyroid function. The thyroid hormones are made from iodine that enters our body through food. We have discussed that in the USA, autoimmune disease is the most common cause of thyroid disorders, but worldwide, the deficiency of iodine deficiency is the main cause of thyroid dysfunction. This has occurred due to the addition of iodine to salt (iodized salt) in the US since the 1920s. Moreover, the consumption of grains, dairy and fish have significantly helped them in maintaining a healthy thyroid gland, as these foods are the best natural source of iodine.

However, deficiency and excess of iodine are damaging to the thyroid gland. One should be very careful in taking iodine supplementation as it can lead to aggravation of symptom in individuals with Hashimoto's disease as it can lead to the overproduction of autoimmune antibodies.

Vitamin B12

Vitamin B12 is the naturally present in cereals, dairy, liver and muscle meat, and in seafood, including salmon and molluscs is beneficial for the thyroid health. Regular use of these food components helps the thyroid to function optimally.

Vitamin D

Vitamin D is a very crucial nutrient and its

deficiency has been found to be linked to thyroid dysfunction and Hashimoto's disease. It has been found that around 90% of individuals who are suffering from Hashimoto's disease were deficient in vitamin D. However, it is yet to be determined that the low vitamin D levels were the cause of Hashimoto's or were caused by the disease.

Hyperthyroidism has been linked with low vitamin D levels in the body. Graves' disease has been known to cause bone loss which leads to a deficiency of vitamin D. The treatments of hyperthyroidism generally involve the use of vitamin D supplements that help in regaining the bone mass that has been lost due to hormonal imbalance.

Some of the best food sources of vitamin D include milk, include fatty fish, dairy, mushrooms and eggs. Sunlight is considered as one of the greatest sources of vitamin D, but this source is influenced by the altitude, equatorial location and the season. So, one should keep a balance between vitamin D supplement and sun exposure to get the required amount of vitamin D.

Selenium

Selenium is an essential mineral and is involved in various metabolic processes in the body, including the immune system, fertility, cognitive abilities and longevity. It has been found that the thyroid gland has the highest concentration of selenium. It is a vital component of the enzymes present in the thyroid gland that help in the normal functioning of the thyroid.

Research has shown that selenium has significant effects on thyroid antibody titers and on general wellbeing in patients with Hashimoto's. Selenium can be obtained by utilizing, selenium-rich foods, for example, Brazil nuts, and seafood including tuna, lobster and crab.

Vitamin B12

Vitamin B12 is the naturally present in cereals, dairy, liver and muscle meat, and in seafood, including salmon and molluscs is beneficial for the thyroid health. Regular use of these food components helps the thyroid to function optimally.

High Protein Intake

Proteins are an important part of our diet and body. It has been found that proteins help increase the metabolic rate of the body. Individuals with hypothyroidism have experienced benefit by increasing their protein intake. Various researches show that higher-protein diet aids in increasing the rate of metabolism in the body and hence helps with symptoms of hypothyroidism.

Exercise

Good physical activity and an active lifestyle are important determinants of our health. Various thyroid disorders have been known to be positively controlled by yoga and exercises. Being physically active have been shown significant results in managing symptoms of hypothyroid, including fatigue, weight gain and depression. Similarly, individuals suffering from hyperthyroidism have reported being able to manage their symptoms in a better way by being physically active and exercising in routine. Exercise has shown positive results in regulating sleep disorders, anxiety and muscular pain experienced by hyperthyroid patients. Exercise helps improve the metabolism of the body and boost various metabolic processes in the cell. It helps the body to remain active and fight off fatigue and anxiety, which are major symptoms of Graves' disease. Research shows that by following simple yoga exercises, one can manage thyroid disorders in a better way.

The link between Hypothyroidism and Exercise

As we already know that the thyroid hormone functions to regulate the speed of metabolism. And people with a faster metabolism, tend to burn more calories even while resting, as compared to individuals with a slow metabolism. Individuals suffering hypothyroidism tend to make less amount of thyroid hormone, which leads to a slower metabolism and they burn fewer calories at rest.

There are various health risk and complications associated with a slow metabolism. These include fatigue, weakness, increased level of blood cholesterol, and difficulty in losing weight. Exercise helps people with hypothyroid to boost their metabolism and helps them manage their symptoms in a better way. Special high-intensity cardio, including brisk walk, running, rowing and hiking are the recommended exercises for the individual with hypothyroidism

5.1 Foods that are Bad for Thyroid Function

Goitrogens

Goitrogens are obtained from vegetables, such as cabbage, cauliflower and broccoli where they are present in the form goitrin. When goitrin is hydrolyzed, it releases goitrogens. It has been found that goitrin inhibits the production of thyroid hormones. But only in individuals who have an iodine deficiency. Soy is also a potent source of goitrogen, and it is advised to take these vegetables in cooked form and in a checked amount to avoid its negative effects on the thyroid functions.

Millet, a grain that has much nutritious value and is part of the diet of people all over the world has been found to have anti-thyroid activity. It hinders with the production of thyroid hormones even in individuals without iodine deficiency. Individuals with thyroid dysfunction are asked to replace millet with some other grain.

People suffering from any kind of thyroid disorders should avoid certain green vegetables, including Russian kale, broccoli rabe, collards, brussels sprouts, cauliflower, broccoli and cabbage. These vegetables also have numerous health benefits and hypothyroid individuals can enjoy the benefits if they consume this food in a moderate amount and avoid excessive consumption.

Gluten

Hypothyroidism has been found to be linked with an underlying autoimmune disorder, which can lead to other complications. That is why hypothyroid individuals are considered to be at a higher risk of developing other autoimmune disorders, such as celiac disease. Gluten acts as a major trigger of celiac disease and individual who are allergic to this protein develop chronic inflammation in the small intestine. Studies support the idea that people with thyroid hormonal disorder should avoid ingestion of gluten to protect their immune system. Gluten is present in barley, rye, oat and wheat and people with autoimmune-based hypothyroidism should cut gluten out of their diets to check if their condition might improve.

Soy

Studies have highlighted the role of soy as a deregulator of the thyroid gland. Soy proteins interfere with the process of thyroid hormone production. In a case study, a woman developed severe hypothyroidism after consuming soy-based health drink. And her symptoms improved with taking thyroid hormone medications and stop consuming the drink. So, it is advisable for hypothyroid patients to avoid soy-based food and consume them in very little amount. Major food sources of soy include edamame, soy sauce, tofu, miso and soymilk.

Processed Food

Hypothyroid individuals should take special care of their diet and calorie intake. It is highly recommended that they avoid processed food that are very high in calories and low in nutrition. Consumption of such food can cause weight gain and aggravate other symptoms of thyroid dysfunction. Some of the most common processed foods include cakes, hot dogs, doughnuts, fast food and cookies.

5.2 Complete Diet Plan for Managing Hypothyroidism

It is a fact that diet cannot cure hypothyroidism. But it can help to manage the symptoms of thyroid disorders in the following three ways:

- Consumption of nutritious foods that promote the health of thyroid glands such as zinc, iodine, and selenium should be promoted. Iodine rich food includes cheese, ice cream, milk, seafood, eggs and iodized salts. Food that is a good source of selenium includes beef, turkey, Brazil nut, eggs, shrimp, tuna and ham. And the best sources of zinc include chicken, oysters, beef, crab, legumes, yoghurt and fortified cereal.
- Avoid consumption of foods that interfere with normal thyroid function, including soy and goitrogens, can improve symptoms of hypothyroidism
- Being cautious while taking certain supplements and foods that may interfere with the absorption of thyroid hormone during replacement therapy.

It is recommended that an individual with hypothyroidism should maintain a balanced diet that contains plenty of vegetables, fruits, proteins, and a moderate amount of good carbohydrates. A general diet plan for a person with hypothyroidism is given below:

- Breakfast: Eggs scrambled with cheese and gluten-free or whole-wheat toast OR oatmeal berries with yoghurt and mushrooms or banana or pineapple smoothie
- Lunch: Salad with grilled chicken or grilled shrimp
- Dinner: Beef stir-fry or baked salmon with vegetables and brown rice OR roasted beans with grilled seafood topped with peppers and pineapples

5.3 Complete Diet Plan for Managing Hyperthyroidism

The symptoms of hyperthyroidism can be managed through a cautious diet and healthy eating. In the next section, we will include the diet that should be followed by hyperthyroid patients and what food should be avoided to decrease the intensity of related symptoms.

Low-iodine foods

Iodine is metabolized by the thyroid gland to make thyroid hormones. It is recommended to take a low-iodine diet which aids to reduce the level of thyroid hormones. Some of the common food items that need to be replaced by regular one that has high iodine content include coffee or tea without dairy or soy-based creamers, egg whites, non-iodized salts, unsalted nuts, unsalted butter, popcorn without iodized salt, oats, potatoes, organic homemade bread without salt, eggs and dairy.

Cruciferous vegetables, including broccoli, cabbage, bamboo shoots, cassava, mustard, kale and cauliflower should be included in the diet as they decrease the production of thyroid hormone by the thyroid gland.

Iron

Iron is essential for various vital functions of the body, including regulation of thyroid health. Deficiency of iron has been linked to hyperthyroidism. That is why it is advised that we obtain enough iron through our diet by consuming the following foods:

- Nuts
- Red meat

- Dried beans
- Lentils
- Chicken and Turkey
- Whole grains
- Green leafy vegetables

Selenium

Food rich in selenium- are helpful in balancing and regulating the levels of thyroid hormone and protect the thyroid from various dysfunctions. Some of the best sources of selenium include tea, chia seeds, rice, beef meat, lamb meat, mushrooms, chicken, turkey, sunflower seeds and oat bran.

Zinc

Zinc is an essential mineral that regulates the immune system and thyroid health. The best sources of zinc include mushrooms, beef meat, chickpeas, cocoa powder, lamb meat, and cashews.

Calcium and vitamin D

The bones and joints of individuals with hyperthyroidism become weak and brittle and there is the loss of bone mass due to the imbalance of thyroid hormone. Vitamin D and calcium supplement an important part of the treatment of hyperthyroidism as they function to restore healthy bones. The best sources of calcium include kale, white beans, calcium-fortified orange juice, collard greens, almond milk, beef liver, vitamin-D fortified cereals, mushrooms, and spinach.

Good Fats

Fats that are obtained from whole organic whole foods and unprocessed play an important role in the reduction of inflammation from the body. Th provides protection to the thyroid gland that produces thyroid hormones in a balanced amount. Nondairy fats are an essential part of a low-iodine diet, which include, unsalted seeds and nuts, coconut oil, avocado oil, flaxseed oil, sunflower oil, olive oil and safflower oil.

Herbs and Spices

Studies have shown that certain herbs and spices have anti-inflammatory properties. This property aid in reducing inflammation from the body and protects the thyroid gland from dysfunction. We can easily include them in our food to get both antioxidation benefits and flavour to it. Some of the most useful spices and herbs for managing hyperthyroidism include black pepper, turmeric, and green chillies.

Avoid the use of Excess Iodine

Hyperthyroidism can be controlled if one can cut down the intake of high-iodine food products. Some tips in this respect are given below

- Avoid the use of seafood and seafood additives, such as sushi, seaweed, lobster, algae, prawns, and crabs.
- Avoid milk and dairy that have high iodine content, including cheese, salted butter, etc.
- Avoid egg yolk.
- Avoid using iodized water and food colouring.
- Avoid using gluten and soy-based food products.
- There are some medications that contain iodine. It is recommended to avoid the use of such medications. These include various cough syrups, amiodarone, herbal supplements, vitamin mixtures, and medical contrast dyes.

Nitrates

Certain salts such as nitrates increase the absorption process of iodine by the thyroid gland which leads to overproduction of thyroid hormone. This can be avoided by taking special care while consuming certain food that has high nitrate content. These include spinach, celery, processed meat including pepperoni, sausage, salami and bacon, leeks, fennel cabbage, parsley, carrot, turnip, pumpkin, cabbage, and beets.

Caffeine

Studies show that the use of caffeine can exacerbate the symptoms of hyperthyroidism, such as anxiety, irritability, nervousness, trouble breathing and increase heart rate. Certain foods and beverages are the primary sources of caffeine, such as tea, coffee, chocolate, and soda. If you experience these symptoms on the consumption of caffeine, it is advised to stop using any caffeine-based products and look for healthier alternatives such as vitamin water, flavoured green herbal tea, and hot apple cider.

5.4 Lifestyle Changes for Hypothyroidism

Individuals with hypothyroidism have a high tendency to gain weight and are at high risk of developing cardiovascular and metabolic disorders, including hypertension and diabetes. Due to the complex nature of thyroid hormone disorders, the mere use of medications for its management is not enough. That is why thyroid and other hormonal disorder require a certain change in lifestyle, that involves what we eat, do, and think.

Various studies have highlighted the role of lifestyle in the manifestation as well as management of hypothyroidism. Some of the most important tips that have significant effects in controlling thyroid hormone levels in the body and maintaining a healthy weight are given below:

Diet

Individuals with hypothyroid should include low to moderate carbs levels in their diet. This allows them to maintain a healthy weight. They should avoid a ketogenic diet, which has much fewer carbs as it may further decrease the levels of thyroid hormone in the body.

Relax and Rest

It is recommended to take around 7–8 hours of sleep at night. This allows the body to heal and improve metabolic rate.

Mindful eating

This means we should pay attention to what we are and eating, why we are eating it. This practice allows us to develop a relationship with the food we are eating, and it helps the body to metabolize it in a better and efficient way. For hypothyroid individuals, it is a big plus as it mindful eating helps them in losing weight.

Practice yoga or Meditation

Yoga and meditation play a major role in helping us de-stress and enhances our health and wellbeing. Research has shown that yoga helps to improve the metabolism of the body which protects from unwanted weight gain.

Use Herbal Supplements

It is recommended to take some alternative medicines, such as herbal medicines to help manage the symptoms of hypothyroidism in a better way. Researches have shown that certain herbs, including ashwagandha (*Withania somnifera*), Gotu kola (*Centella asiatica*), and coleus (*Coleus forskohlii*) help with symptoms of hypothyroidism.

6-Thyroid Medications, Do's and Don'ts

There are several medications that are being used for the treatment of thyroid disorders. However, in order to gain full benefits of the medication, one should keep certain things under check as thyroid medications tend to interact with various food components and supplements and can lose their efficacy. Some of the main points that need to be taken under special consideration include:

- Calcium supplements can interfere with the absorption process of thyroid medications, that is why it is important that patients must take calcium supplements and thyroid medications with around four hours gap.
- Coffee decreases the absorption of thyroid medications, so a gap of at least two hours should be placed between the two.
- Fibre supplements also interfere with the absorption of thyroid medication so medication should be taken at least four hours

before or after the use of such supplements.
- Chromium picolinate which is used for weight loss and control of blood sugar can decrease the absorption of thyroid medications, so proper time gap should be given by individuals taking both medications
- Flavonoids that are naturally present in various vegetables, fruits, and tea have been shown to interfere with thyroid functions. Therefore, special care should be taken while taking flavonoid supplements together with thyroid medications to get the best results of both.

7-Genetic and Environmental Basis of Thyroid Dysfunction

Thyroid dysfunctions are complex and are caused by various underlying genetic and environmental factors. Hormonal imbalance of any kind becomes a syndrome rather than a disease as it can affect various cellular functions in different parts of the body. Various thyroid disorders, especially those that result due to autoimmune dysfunction are considered to have multiple extrinsic factors that may trigger the autoimmune response. Moreover, this autoimmune response is more likely to occur in individuals who are genetically predisposed to the disease. Research shows that various nutritive factors (intrinsic factors) and pollutants present in the environment (extrinsic factors) together lead to thyroid dysfunction. It has been found that the presence of various environmental pollutants, including pesticides and organochlorines, act as a major trigger for thyroid disorders.

However, more research is required to understand the genetic factors that are considered as risk factors for the development of thyroid dysfunction. In the next section, we will focus on the genetic aspect of this disease and try to find the link between hypothyroidism, hyperthyroidism, immune system disorder and related genes.

7.1 Genetics and Thyroid Disorder

Thyroid hormone is a vast acting hormone. It plays a significant role in maintaining human physiology and regulate all tissues of the body in one way or another. Thyroid hormones have an impact on the growth and development, cognitive abilities, bone health, cardiovascular function, metabolism and balance of energy. In recent years, the key role of genetics in normal and abnormal thyroid function has come under the limelight. This has improved our knowledge about the complexities of thyroid hormone action, the variations between individuals and the resulting disease, that is responsible for variation in clinical phenotypes.

7.2 Common Genetic Variation

Genetic variations are caused by the presence of SNPs (single nucleotide polymorphisms) that account for 90% of the variations that are present across the human genome. The genetic studies that have been focused on finding the link between the thyroid phenotypes and the underlying genes have used methods like, whole genome sequencing and genome-wide association studies (GWAS). These studies have shown that some genes, such as that of TSH receptor and thyroglobulin, seem to have an important role in the manifestation of autoimmune thyroid disease.

The genetic variations in the genes responsible for thyroid dysfunction are manifested as variation in the levels of circulating free thyroxine (T4), TSH and free tri-iodothyronine (T3) among different individuals with thyroid dysfunction. These genetic variations have different phenotypic effects such as changes in mood, cholesterol levels, and longevity. This shows that various genes control the thyroid function and they are also involved in the regulation of other metabolic changes in the body.

Various genes have been found to be linked with the development of autoimmune disorder that affects the thyroid gland. Many genes have been identified that are associated with Hashimoto's thyroiditis in a unique wat. For example, the genetic variant MTRR+66AA is more common in people that have severe Hashimotos's thyroiditis as compared to those individuals who show mild symptoms of the disease. This gene is involved in the epigenetic control of gene expression and carries out the methylation of DNA. The variant of this gene encodes methionine synthase reductase (MTRR) that have altered abilities to methylate DNA.

DNA methylation is a mechanism that cells utilize to carry out the regulation of the gene expression, usually for turning them off. Defects in DNA methylation is considered an important factor in autoimmune thyroid disease. And these epigenetic changes play a significant role in the development of autoimmune disorders, such as Graves' disease and Hashimoto's thyroiditis.

7.3 Genetics of Thyroid Function

The heritability studies have shown that a major proportion of free T4, free T3, and TSH variation is genetically derived. There are three main genes that are responsible for this variation and the polymorphisms within these genes have been shown to be linked with thyroid function. These genes include iodothyronine deiodinase 1 (DIO1), phosphodiesterase 8B (PDE8B), and F-actin-capping protein subunit beta (CAPZB).

Furthermore, a polymorphism in the TSH receptor gene (TSHR) has been shown to be linked with thyroid function in different population-based studies. Several other genes have been proposed to be linked with thyroid function but there is not enough mapping data available for these genes or these genes might be incompatible for life. The function of the thyroid hormones and their interaction at the genetic levels are given in Figure 4.

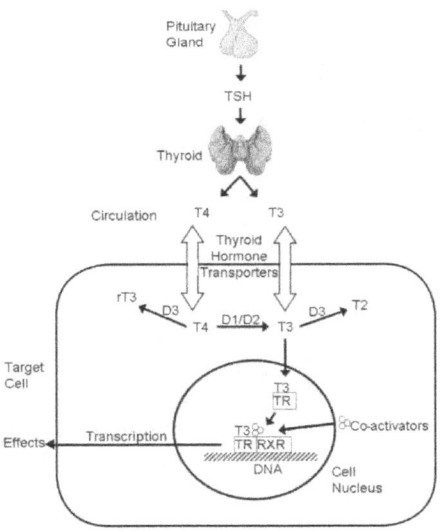

Figure 4. The thyroid hormones and their genetic regulation

7.4 Variation in Thyroid Genes and Their Clinical Manifestations

There are only a few genes that have been identified so far that are involved in the direct manifestation of thyroid disorder. It is a fact that the final concentration of T3 in the cells is influenced by many factors that can alter the binding of T3 to TR, resulting in low thyroid levels in the body. So, it may happen that the thyroid function is normal but the receptors in the cell are defective. Studies have shown that the three genes that are mutated in thyroid disorders are also linked with various our abnormalities and disease. They are given in Table 1.

Table 1. List of thyroid-related genes that are linked with various clinical phenotypes

Gene	SNP	Phenotype
DIO2	rs225014/rs12885300	Osteoarthritis
	rs225010/rs225012	Mental retardation in iodine deficient areas
	rs225014	Psychological well-being on T4
	rs225014	Preference for T3/T4 over T4 therapy
	rs225014/rs12885300	Bipolar affective disorder
	rs225014	*Hypertension/blood pressure*
TSHR	rs1991517	Bone density
	rs1991517	Insulin resistance
	rs10149689/rs12050077	Longevity
OATP1C1	rs10770704	*Psychological well-being on T4*
DIO1	rs11206244/rs12095080	IGF-1

8-Nutrigenomics and Thyroid Disease

As described earlier, thyroid dysfunction is a syndrome as it is very complex and has complicated effects on the body. Moreover, the complex interactions between the genes involved, epigenetics, and triggering of autoimmune diseases like Hashimoto's thyroiditis have made the disease very hard to understand and predict. However, the fact that epigenetic regulation through DNA methylation is present as a major cause of thyroid dysfunction suggests a prospect for nutrigenomics to regulate an individual's risk of developing the condition.

Nutrigenomics involves the interaction of nutrients present in our diet with our genes. This branch of genetics has gained special attention in recent decades where such interactions have proved to be beneficial for the prevention and treatment of various diseases. Food is considered an important part of epigenetic regulation as there are some bioactive nutrients that alter the DNA function and thus the gene expression. Epigenetics has opened new horizons to understand and manage thyroid dysfunction and many bioavailable nutrients have been studied and are part of treatment therapies for thyroid disorders. DNA methylation is primarily dependent on an adequate supply of bioavailable nutrients including vitamin B and folate. Other nutritional factors have been identified as possible candidates for the role in regulating the risk or progression of autoimmune conditions. Some of these nutrients are described below.

❖ **Vitamin B and Folate**

vitamins B2, B6, and B12, folate, betaine, choline, and methionine are considered vital bioactive nutrients. They are needed for the production of S-adenosylmethionine (SAMe), which acts as a donor for methyl groups in the DNA methylation process. Insufficient levels of these nutrients in the diet lead to decreased production of low SAMe and the process of DNA methylation is halted. The decrease in the methylation process increases the risk of autoimmune conditions. Polymorphisms such as MTHFR variants and MTRR variants affect folate metabolism also affects the process of DNA methylation and increase the risk of autoimmune thyroid disorder (AITD).

Taking a good nutritious diet with a sufficient amount of vitamin B and folate ensures that we get the required level of methyl donors. This allows the body to function optimally and one can enjoy a robust and healthy life. folate and other B vitamins have been directly linked with improvement in thyroid function and enhancement in immune system activity.

❖ Vitamin D

Vitamin D is a very important nutrient that should be part of our diet. Studies have increasingly implicated vitamin D in the development of autoimmune conditions. And it has been found that the active form of vitamin D, 1,25(OH)2D, controls the expression of around 200 genes. Most of these genes are involved in the regulation of the immune system. Various studies have found that deficiency of vitamin D deficiency is more common in individuals with autoimmune thyroid disease (AITD). In a study, it was reported that around 72% of AITD patients were vitamin D deficient, compared to the healthy controls. In another study, more than 90% of people with Hashimoto's disease had vitamin D insufficiency as compared to the control.

❖ Selenium

Selenium plays a significant role in thyroid health and can be considered as the most essential nutrient for the optimum production of thyroid hormones. This trace mineral is part of the amino acid selenocysteine (Sec) which is a key component of a group of proteins known as selenoproteins.

These proteins are a family of important antioxidant enzymes. These include glutathione peroxidase (GPx), thioredoxin reductase (TrxR), and iodothyronine deiodinases (DIO). DIO enzymes are involved in the regulation of metabolism and control the activity of thyroid hormones thyroxine (T4), and (T3). Selenoproteins also regulate oxidative and inflammatory processes in the body. The level of selenoproteins vary greatly among individuals and is different in different ethnic and geographic population. An optimum level of Se in the cell is essential for the maintenance of homeostasis.

Nutrigenetic studies have shown that different Se levels in the diet are required for different individuals, depending on the genetic variants. The effective dietary Se intake for one individual is different from that for others. That is why it is important that one should keep check of their selenoproteins levels and then formulate an appropriate diet plan for the optimum intake of selenium. And like other micronutrients, the suboptimal intake level of Se may lead to the development of various chronic diseases and too high Se level have been associated with toxicity.

Selenium is considered important for thyroid functions. Recent studies have shown that the essential trace element selenium is present in the form of selenocysteine in all three deiodinases that regulate the thyroid function. These findings suggest that a clear-cut link is present between selenium and thyroid function. And the thyroid contains more selenium than any other tissue and that selenium deficiency aggravates the manifestation of endemic myxedematous cretinism and autoimmune thyroid disease.

9-Oxidative Stress and Thyroid Dysfunction

Research has shown that oxidative stress is one of the most important triggers of hypothyroidism. Hypothyroidism is also defined as the state of increased oxidative stress. Oxidative stress is caused due to an imbalance between the antioxidant defence systems and the rate of reactive oxygen species (ROS) production. It causes various physiological changes in the cell, including lipid peroxidation and oxidative DNA damage. It also interferes with intracellular signal transduction pathways and compromises the endocrine system. These change in the intracellular redox status causes activation of protein kinases, such as, tyrosine kinase, and protein kinase C, that leads to altered cellular functions.

As described earlier, the thyroid hormones (THs) effect at the cellular level by binding to specialized receptors that couple to both genomic and nongenomic signalling pathways. These hormones undergo transformations in the peripheral tissues, mainly in the form of deiodination. The main metabolic effect of thyroid hormones is the acceleration of the basal metabolism rate 'both catabolic and anabolic. This leads to an increased expenditure of energy, increased oxygen consumption, elevated respiratory rate, and more heat production.

Thyroid hormones also influence cell antioxidant status. Hypothyroidism-linked oxidative stress is caused by both increased production of free radicals and reduced efficiency of the antioxidative defence. The excessive production of thyroid-stimulating hormone (TSH) leads to an alteration in the oxidative stress processes. As the hypothyroidism-induced dysfunction of the mitochondrial respiratory chain leads to the increased production of free radicals.

Lipid peroxidation— a trademark of oxidative stress—is increased in hyperlipidemia, which is a primary symptom of hypothyroidism. The presence of oxidative stress in hypothyroidism associates with the risk f of developing atherosclerosis. Various metabolic disorders that are caused by autoimmune-induced hypothyroidism can increase oxidative stress. Chronic inflammation can lead to endothelial dysfunction and reduces the availability of nitric oxide (NO) which leads to increased oxidative stress in Hashimoto's thyroiditis.

Oxidative stress can damage the thyroid gland in the presence of iodine excess. It has been reported that iodide stimulates the generation of hydrogen peroxide in thyroid slices and that leads to the apoptosis of thyroid cells at very high concentrations.

Various research supports the role of the use of antioxidant supplements to control the oxidative stress caused by thyroid dysfunction. In a study, the MDA levels were monitored in the body, as they are considered as the oxidative stress biomarker. It was found that in hypothyroid patients, the level of MDA levels is quite high. After subsequent treatment with antioxidant, L-thyroxine, the stress marker reduced to a significant level and the condition of the patient also improved. Moreover, selenium has been found to acts as a cofactor for the TH deiodinases that activate and then deactivate various thyroid hormones and their metabolites. Selenium has the ability to stop the progression of thyroid autoimmunity.

9.1 Effects of Oxidative Stress on Thyroid Gland

Oxidative stress has been associated with both

hyperthyroidism and hypothyroidism. However, the mechanisms which lead to the generation of oxidative stress is different in the two clinical conditions of thyroid disorder. These mechanisms are given below:

- Increased production of ROS in hyperthyroidism
- Decreased availability of antioxidants in hypothyroidism

A model of the interrelationships between oxidative stress, inflammation, and thyroid derangement is given in figure 5. Inflammation that is caused by hormone and cytokine, such as leptin, TNF-alpha, etc., leads to increased oxidative stress in the body. This oxidative stress affects the function of thyroid function that leads to various physiological changes in the body. At the tissue level, hypothyroidism adds to the oxidative stress, which worsens the symptoms of hypothyroidism by inhibiting the function of deiodinases.

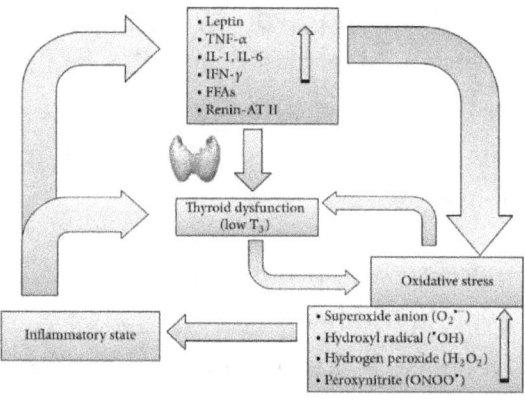

Figure 5. The effects of oxidative stress on thyroid functions

9.2 The Best Antioxidant Diet for Controlling Thyroid Dysfunctions

Nature has provided us with powerful antioxidants. The use of these antioxidant nutrients can help us manage the oxidative stress levels in the body. Individuals with thyroid dysfunction can greatly benefit by including certain foods in their diets. Some of the most widely studied antioxidants that have proven benefits of antioxidants are discussed below:

- Blueberries
- Pumpkins
- Oatmeal (Gluten-free)
- Organic eggs
- Beans

- Brazil nuts
- Red bell peppers
- Dark Chocolate
- Sardines

Blueberries are very rich in nutrients and are loaded with fibre. They are an excellent source of vitamin c, manganese, vitamin K, and antioxidants. By adding blueberries in our diet, we can get various benefits, as it helps lower the blood pressure, control the level of cholesterol, boost our brain function and fights cancer.

Pumpkin is an excellent source of antioxidants, along with zinc, fibre, vitamin C, Vitamin A, magnesium, and potassium. They also are a good source of L tryptophan, which is a chemical compound that promotes the feelings of well-being. This helps in managing depression. Pumpkin is also anti-inflammatory, and it can help with joint pain, organ functions and relieve stress from the body.

Oatmeal (gluten-free) oatmeal is the best option for a gluten-free diet. This is ideal for people with hypothyroidism as they suffer from gluten intolerance. Oatmeal provides energy to the body as it is a good body, provides healthy fibre, and enhances the immune system. It is also known to maintain blood sugar levels.

Organic eggs are also a good source of antioxidants. They contain high levels of tyrosine and tryptophan and can reduce the level of oxidative stress in the body. This antioxidative effect provides a protective effect against cardiovascular diseases and cancer. These eggs are also enriched with nine essential amino acids, vitamin A, vitamin E, vitamin B2, vitamin B5, iron, sulfur, and omega-3 fatty acids.

Red bell peppers are an excellent source of antioxidants, and also provide vitamin E, vitamin C, manganese, and various vital carotenoids. Adding red bell pepper helps us improve the spice level of our food along with nutritious values.

Sardines are an excellent source of protein and provide us with various amino acids. They are strong antioxidants and are also rich in omega-3 fatty acids, vitamin B12 and vitamin D. Sardines are a good source of vitamin B12, and vitamin D. They are also rich in protein, which provides us with amino acids.

Brazil nuts are a good source of vitamin B, Vitamin E, folates, thiamin, copper, riboflavin, niacin, calcium, manganese, potassium, selenium and iron. Selenium deficiency is very common in hypothyroidism patients. Just adding two brazil nuts to our daily diet fulfils the recommended daily dose of selenium.

Natural, unprocessed cacao, dark chocolate is an excellent antioxidant. It is also rich in zinc, manganese, iron, magnesium, and calcium. The cocoa powder or chocolate we buy from stores is full of additives, including sweeteners, so that is not much recommended.

10- Problems related to Thyroid diseases and Their Treatment via Diet

10.1 Thyroid Disorder and Depression

Thyroid hormones have a significant effect on our mood and thought processes. As other hormones that determine our feelings and attitude towards things and situations, thyroid hormones also play a central role in the way we feel. The link between thyroid function and behavioural and mood disorders has been recognized since long. Historically, this link was first established around 200 years ago and in 1825, it was reported that there is a connection between thyroid disorder and nervous affectations. Today, it has been widely recognized that disruptions in thyroid function may substantially affect emotion and cognition and alter the mental status in a negative way.

The deficiency and excessiveness of thyroid hormones, both, can lead to mood abnormalities, which mainly includes depression. Such depression is generally reversible with proper thyroid treatment. However, this relation acts in both way and studies have shown that depression can lead to y slight thyroid dysfunction, but an acute thyroid disorder is rare. Individuals with hypothyroidism and hyperthyroidism show symptoms of depression. A systematic review (2018) reported that people with Hashimoto's disease are more likely to develop depression and anxiety as compared to controls. It was found that around 24% of the test subjects experienced depression and nearly 42% suffered from anxiety.

10.1.1 Thyroid Hormone Metabolism in the Brain

As we know that there is a complex interplay of hormones and enzymes at the hypothalamic-pituitary-thyroid axis (HPT). Various factors, including thyroid hormones, thyroid receptors, deiodinase enzymes, and transporter proteins interact with each other in an intricate manner to maintain energy balance in the body. The thyroid hormones are regulated by pituitary thyrotropin (TSH) which itself is fueled by hypothalamic thyrotropin-releasing hormone and downregulated by high levels of serum thyroid hormones. The understanding of these interactions is considered vital for understanding the pathophysiology of psychiatric disorders related to thyroid hormone and to elucidate the proper treatment.

10.1.2 Thyroid Dysfunction and Related Neuropsychiatric Disorders

Hypothyroidism and hyperthyroidism can lead to the manifestation of various neuropsychiatric symptoms, which can range from mild depression and anxiety to severe psychosis. The most common neuropsychiatric effects of thyroid dysfunction include anxiety, dysphoria, lack of concentration, irritability, and emotional lability. In elderly patients, however, thyroid dysfunction is manifested as mimicking a depressive disorder that includes dementia, lethargy, and apathy. The most common neuropsychological effects of thyroid dysfunction are anxiety disorders that affect around 60% of patients with hyperthyroid, followed by depression, which occurs in 31 to 69% of hyperthyroid individuals.

Hypothyroid patients are more likely to suffer from depression, cognitive dysfunction, psychomotor slowing, and apathy as a result of thyroid dysfunction. In cases of severe hypothyroidism, clinical symptoms may manifest as dementia and severe depression.

The rule here is simple, too much thyroid hormone makes your metabolism fast, makes you anxious. While too little of the energy hormone makes you slow and depressed. American Association of Clinical Endocrinologists believes that the diagnosis of hypothyroidism must be considered in every patient who is suffering from depression. As among the various neurophysiological manifestations of thyroid disorders, depression is the most prevalent.

10.1.3 Thyroid Hormone Status in Patients with Depression

Several thyroid abnormalities have been associated with mood disorders particularly depression. However, most patients with depression do not have biochemical evidence of thyroid dysfunction. Thyroid abnormalities are clinically determined through various tests that may show low T3 levels, elevated T4 levels, increased rT3, reduced TSH response to TRH, presence of antithyroid antibodies, and increased cerebrospinal fluid (CSF) TRH concentrations. However, a special situation that is termed as brain hypothyroidism occurs in some cases where the level of thyroid hormone in the brain is disturbed as compared to the peripheral thyroid hormones and is marked by a low level of

CSF TTR in individuals with depression.

10.1.4 Thyroid Hormone Supplementation in Depression

The use of thyroid hormone supplements for the treatment of thyroid-linked depression has been known since the 1960s. The T3 hormone has been considered as an effective antidepressant and various meta-analysis of trials have shown positive results in relieving the symptoms of depression in patients who use tricyclic antidepressants. Recently, the use of selective serotonin reuptake inhibitors (SSRIs) in combination with T3 for the treatment of refractory depression have shown confounding results.

There are various clinically used versions and variants of thyroid hormones for the treatment of depression and other neuropsychological disorders related to thyroid dysfunction. Some of them are given below:

- Levothyroxine is the most used drug for the treatment of thyroid-related depression. It is a purified form of the synthetic T4 hormone. Levothyroxine works in the same way as the thyroid hormone. It is well absorbed in the body and provides stable levels of the hormone.

- Other options of drugs that are used to treat depression and anxiety include liothyronine (Cytomel), which is a synthetic version of T3.

10.1.5 Treating Thyroid-related Depression with Diet

Among the various effects of thyroid dysfunction, the increase in oxidative stress, especially in the brain, can lead to the manifestation of symptoms of depression and anxiety. Thyroid dysfunction can be managed through diet and research has shown that by adding proper nutrients to our diet we can cope with various behavioural disorders and can improve our mood. Some of the most powerful antioxidants that are present in the diet that can help us manage thyroid-induced depression are given below:

❖ **Vitamin E**

Vitamin E is a very potent antioxidant and is found in wheat, nuts, seeds and vegetable oil. Vitamin C is present in high amounts in oranges, blueberries, kiwi, grapefruits, strawberries, tomatoes potatoes, and broccoli. One can easily add these foods to the diet and can get amazing benefits.

❖ **Beta-carotene**

This antioxidant is present in peaches, pumpkins,

carrots, apricot, spinach, and sweet potato.

❖ Good Carbs

The use of good or smart carbohydrates in our diet has e been found to have a calming effect. Such carbohydrates mediate the release of serotonin, which is the mood-enhancing chemical produced in the brain. The reduction of serotonin is linked with depression and feeling of distress, which can be reduced by adding good carbohydrates in our diet.

❖ Protein-Rich Foods

Research has shown that taking a protein-based diet makes us more alert and active. By adding proteins in our diet, we can cope with depression and fatigue. The foods that are a good source of proteins include tuna, turkey, and chicken. They contain the amino acid tryptophan, which is the precursor of serotonin. Other foods that are excellent sources of protein include milk, yoghurt, poultry, peas, beans, fish, cheese and soy products. People with thyroid disorders should take protein several times a day, to clear their minds and boost their energy levels.

❖ Thyroid Disorder and Fatigue

The thyroid gland regulates the metabolic rate of the body and determines how active and fresh we feel. The dysregulation of the thyroid hormone results in undesired changes in the metabolism that negatively affects our energy levels. And that is why individuals with thyroid disorder suffer from a constant state of feeling tired and fatigued. Fatigue is a state of relentless exhaustion and debilitating tiredness that does not go away by resting and makes you deprived of carrying out your daily activities. Individuals who experience fatigue feel drained of energy and brain fog.

Thyroid hormone plays an important role in providing the necessary energy as well as motivation we need to carry out our daily chores and business. That is why individuals who experience fatigue and tiredness are advised to get their thyroid level check as thyroid dysfunction is one of the most common underlying factors of fatigue. Fatigue and severe exhaustion are considered as indicators s of undiagnosed or improperly treated thyroid disorder. It has been reported that by adjusting the dose of thyroid medication dose by consulting with the doctor, improving the sleep habits, can significantly improve the symptoms of thyroid-related fatigue and can make one live better with the condition. Unfortunately, in some cases, fatigue persists even after thyroid treatment.

❖ Hashimoto's Disease and Fatigue

Fatigue is a universal symptom of hypothyroidism and occurs as a result of the decrease in the production of thyroid hormone. It causes bone-numbing fatigue as the metabolic rates are decreased to an alarming level and cellular energy is very low. Hypothyroidism-related fatigue can develop gradually or can affect the individual suddenly and can cause difficulty in lifting the head off the pillow in the morning. Untreated or insufficiently treated hypothyroidism can cause exhaustion, which has milder effects than fatigue.

❖ Graves' Disease and Fatigue

Fatigue is also associated with hyperthyroidism and it commonly occurs as a result of anxiety, insomnia, sleep deprivation. These and other symptoms of hyperthyroidism including, increased blood pressure and increased heart rate can also leave you feeling fatigued.

10.2.1 Treatment for Thyroid-related Fatigue

The treatment of hypothyroid which leads to a normal level of thyroid hormone in the body can help improve fatigue or can even make it go away. On the other hand, taking the antithyroid drug in large amount for treating hyperthyroid can worsen the symptoms of fatigue. That is why thyroid hormone replacement medication should be taken in a certain dose that helps relieve fatigue and the dose should be adjusted if you are taking the medicine but still feeling fatigued.

10.3 Thyroid Dysfunction and Sleep Disorder

The most common type of sleep disorder that has been found to be linked with thyroid disorder is sleep apnea. This condition is characterized by a brief period of feeling breathless during sleep. People who suffer from this condition wake up during their sleep as their breathing stops and they have to gasp for air to continue breathing. Sleep apnea can cause severe exhaustion, headaches, and fatigue.

Hypothyroidism has been found to be associated with sleep apnea as low levels of thyroid hormone can affect breathing. A systematic review (2016) of studies based on hypothyroidism and sleep apnea reported that 30% of patients with severe hypothyroidism also suffered from obstructive sleep apnea.

10.4 Thyroid Dysfunction and Anemia

Anaemia is linked with hypothyroidism and is considered the first sign of thyroid disorder. It is characterized by a significant decrease in the red blood cell count. The common symptoms of anaemia include dizziness, the pounding of the heart, shortness of breath and fatigue.

10.5 Thyroid Dysfunction and Iron Deficiency

Iron deficiency is considered as a major sign of thyroid disorder. Individuals with hypothyroidism may suffer from iron deficiency which is the cause of fatigue in most cases. Iron deficiency can also lead to anaemia if left untreated. Taking proper treatment for iron deficiency can considerably improve the symptoms of fatigue.

10.6 Lifestyle changes for Coping with Problems Related to Thyroid Dysfunction

It is now a known fact that lifestyle and diet can help us manage various conditions and diseases. We must recognize the problem, look for related patterns and triggers and find a relevant solution to cope with diseases like thyroid disorder and related problems. As we know that being sleep deprived, unrested and poor diet choices act as major triggers of thyroid disorders, it is wise that we make some changes in our lifestyle to manage the disease and live a better life. Some of the most important changes that may help us improve disorders that are related to thyroid dysfunction are given below:

❖ Get Rested

Fatigue and lethargy are the most common problems related to thyroid dysfunction. That is why it is recommended that one should get enough sleep and rest to allow the body to heal and regain its energy. An eight-hour sleep is recommended to get refreshed and to protect the body from symptoms of sleep deprivation. Managing the thyroid levels and getting proper rest can significantly reduce the symptoms of fatigue and lethargy.

❖ Improve Sleep Quality

The quality of sleep is as important as quantity. Good quality sleep involves a deep, sound sleep that is not interrupted and disturbed. Improving the quality of sleep is related to sleep hygiene and involves various factors that help to in getting a good night's sleep. This involves having a comfortable bed and pillows, cosy environment of the room with the right temperature, smell and feel. Moreover, taking non-prescription sleep aid medications, such as melatonin or herbs such as kava kava, and passionflower should be used to improve your sleep. Getting a good amount of deep sleep refreshes your mind and body and you are good to go for the next day with all your energy.

Passionflower is a native flower to the subtropical and tropical sections of the Americas. It has been known to stimulate emotional balance by relaxation of the nervous system as it acts as a natural stress reducer. It is also widely used to reduce anxiety and acts effectively as a natural sleep aid. Several studies have highlighted the role of Kava Kava to reduce feelings of mild anxiety and sleep-related problems of insomnia.

Melatonin is a natural hormone that is produced in the body. It coordinates with the regulating circadian rhythms, which is our natural sleep and wake cycle of 24 hours. Melatonin improves sleep and helps with major depression.

However, it is wise to consult a physician for sleep disorders and anxiety related to thyroid dysfunction before using any herbal or supplements, as some herbs can further worsen the symptoms related to a thyroid disorder.

❖ Diet Change

Diet is a key factor in managing thyroid disorders and related problems, such as fatigue and sleep issues. It is recommended to avoid processed foods, sugar, gluten, caffeine and dairy to manage various thyroid-related problems. The use of iron supplements and multivitamin have been proved to be beneficial for coping with symptoms of anaemia, fatigue, anxiety and other thyroid-related disorder. The use of antioxidants helps to reduce inflammation and oxidative stress in the body that can occur due to an imbalance of thyroid hormone and can cause fatigue and sleep disorder.

❖ Be Physically Active

Exercise is very important for the wellbeing of body and mind. It is recommended that exercising several times a week will help us burn the extra calories, boost our metabolism and help us sleep better at night. Doing brisk walk, running, jogging and high-intensity training are the recommended exercises one should include in their daily regime

❖ Destress and Yoga

Stress negatively affects our health and disturbs out eating and sleeping pattern. It is recommended that we find time to destress, pause and take a break from our hectic routines. This will allow the mind to relax and help the body heal. Yoga and meditation are also very helpful and is recommended by physicians to cope with the problems of fatigue, anxiety and sleep deprivation caused by thyroid dysfunction.

11-Thyroid dysfunction and Pregnancy

Thyroid hormones play a significant role in the normal development of a baby's brain and nervous system. The baby relies on the mother's thyroid hormone during the first trimester, at around 12 weeks the baby's thyroid starts to work on its own and completely relies on its hormone after 18 to 20 weeks. Human chorionic gonadotropin (hCG) and Estrogen are two pregnancy-related hormones that cause increases the measurement of thyroid hormone levels in the blood. Thyroid related problems are difficult to diagnose during pregnancy due to the increase in levels of thyroid hormones that occur in pregnancy and thyroid dysfunctions. Some of the symptoms of hyperthyroidism or hypothyroidism are easier to diagnose and the doctor advises a test for these thyroid disorders.

11.1 Hyperthyroidism in Pregnancy

Some prominent symptoms of hyperthyroidism that occur in normal pregnancies are increasing in heart rate, difficulty in dealing with heat and tiredness. Some other symptoms include irregular heartbeat, hands may shake and undetermined loss of weight or unable to achieve normal weight gain during pregnancy.

During pregnancy, hyperthyroidism is mainly caused by Graves' disease and found in 1 to 4 out of 1000 pregnancies in the United States. This is an autoimmune disorder in which the immune system starts making antibodies that result in the development of much thyroid hormone. This type of antibody is known as thyroid-stimulating immunoglobulin or TSI.

Graves' disease usually appears during pregnancy, but the symptoms start improving during the second and third trimesters. Rarely, hyperthyroidism in pregnancy is related to hyperemesis gravidarum which causes severe nausea and vomiting that results in weight loss and dehydration. According to experts this severe nausea and vomiting are caused by high levels of hCG during early pregnancy. This increased level of hCG can cause the thyroid to make much thyroid hormone which goes away during the second trimester.

11.1.1 Effect of hyperthyroidism on mother and baby

If the hyperthyroidism left untreated it can lead to miscarriage, premature birth, low birth weight, preeclampsia, and thyroid storm.

In newborn babies, an overactive thyroid can lead to a fast heart rate resulting in heart failure, early closing of a soft spot in the baby's skull, poor weight gain, and irritability.

11.1.2 Diagnosis and Treatment of hyperthyroidism in pregnancy

Some blood tests are taken to measure the thyroid hormone level. Mild hyperthyroidism during pregnancy doesn't need any treatment but if hyperthyroidism is linked to hyperemesis gravidarum, one only needs to treat vomits and dehydration.

In severe cases, doctors may prescribe antithyroid medicines that maintain thyroid hormone. Some antithyroid medicines cause side effects like allergic reactions, decreased number of white blood cells in a body or even liver failure in rare cases.

11.2 Hypothyroidism in Pregnancy

Symptoms during hypothyroidism include extreme tiredness, trouble in dealing with cold, muscle cramps, severe constipation and problems with memory or concentration.

Hypothyroidism in pregnancy is often caused by Hashimoto disease which is found in 2 to 3 out of 100 pregnancies. Hashimoto disease is also an autoimmune disorder in which the immune system makes the antibodies that attack the thyroid which causes inflammation and damage that results in making less able to make thyroid hormones.

11.2.1 Effect of hypothyroidism on mother and baby

If severe hypothyroidism is left untreated during pregnancy it can lead to preeclampsia, anaemia, miscarriage, low birth weight and rarely a congestive heart failure.

11.2.2 Diagnosis of hypothyroidism during pregnancy

A doctor will perform some blood tests to measure thyroid hormone levels. The doctor will also check for certain antibodies in blood to see if Hashimoto's disease is causing hypothyroidism.

11.2.3 Treatment of hypothyroidism during pregnancy

The doctor will advise taking levothyroxine, a thyroid hormone medicine that looks the same as T4, one of the hormones that thyroid normally makes. Levothyroxine is safe for the baby and especially important until the baby makes his thyroid hormone. If you are suffering from hypothyroidism before getting pregnant and you are already taking levothyroxine, then increase the dose.

The doctor will test the thyroid hormone level every 4 to 6 weeks during the first trimester and at least once after 30 weeks. The dose will need an adjustment a few times.

11.3 Postpartum Thyroiditis

Postpartum thyroiditis affects only 1 out of 20 women during the first year after delivery and is most common in women having type 1 diabetes. This inflammation causes the stored thyroid hormone to leak out of the thyroid gland. In early-stage this leakage causes the hormone levels to rise in the blood that leads to hyperthyroidism. This lasts up to three months. This makes the thyroid to become underactive. The hypothyroidism lasts up to a year after delivery while in some women hypothyroidism remains forever.

11.4 Diet for coping with Pregnancy-Related Thyroid Dysfunction

During pregnancy, a mother's body copes with different new changes. So, to overcome that changes well-balanced nutrition is required that helps the body to recover. New moms need to take advantage of the time after delivery because the body acts like a sponge and is ready to absorb the maximum natural nutrients it can get. So new mothers should repair and nourish their bodies by eating healing foods. After giving birth start taking a nutrient-dense and whole food-based item. Cold drinks and cold eatables should be avoided at maximum as they weaken the digestive system and may become a reason for stomach pain. The specific nutrients that might be helpful for the overall health of women after having a baby are described below.

Calcium

Calcium plays a very important role as a body heal from birth. It helps in nerve functioning and blood clotting. A breastfeeding mom will need additional calcium because much calcium is drained out of a mother's body through breast milk for the development of the baby's skeletal system. Good calcium is present in dairy products, dark leafy green vegetables and is also available in supplement form.

Iron

Iron is a very essential part of red blood cells. They can carry and consume oxygen in the cells. With iron deficiency, the body will get weak, fatigued and at a greater risk of catching an infection.

Iron is present in red meat, spinach, beans, and egg yolks. If someone is taking iron supplements than adding food that is rich in Vitamin C like tomatoes, oranges, steamed broccoli, and baked potatoes will help the body for better absorption of iron.

Zinc

zinc helps in supporting a healthy immune system. It also supports increasing the cell production, healing of wounds, growth, and repair of tissues.

Zinc-rich foods included red meat, eggs, fish, oysters, legumes, seafood, poultry, whole grain products, black-eyes peas, and miso.

Protein

Taking enough protein will be helpful to rebuild muscles in the body's postpartum. High protein can be found in chicken, fish, beef, nuts, and eggs.

Water

One should try to drink as much fluid as she can. Take fluids like water, fresh juice, and herbal tea rather than coffee or soda. Try to drink 8 to 10 glass of pure water each day. This will help in the production of milk and will prevent the body from getting dehydrated, constipation and clogged milk ducts.

12-Thyroid Disfunction and Hair Loss

Both conditions of thyroid disorder cause many effects on health. Some of the major effects of thyroid hormone imbalance are discussed below:

12.1 Relationship between Thyroid and Hair

If thyroid disease left untreated, it affects the hairs badly. But before knowing the conditions that cause hair loss one must know how the hair grows. The growth of the hair starts from the root right in the bottom of the hair follicle on the scalp. The roots are fed through blood vessels that help the creation of more cells and ultimately make the hair grow. Then hair comes out of the skin that passes through the oil glands making it soft and shiny. Hairs grow for a short time but then fall out quickly as the regrowth cycle begins.

When the production is disturbed, especially T3 and T4 hormones, the other processes in the body also get affected. Its main effect is on the development of hair at the root. When the hairs fall out, they are not replaced by new growth which results in thinning across your scalp and other areas such as eyebrows.

Another condition which is known as alopecia, which is an autoimmune condition, is often observed in disrupted thyroid conditions which causes hair loss in patches in more distinct areas. With time, this condition may result in baldness. Hairs are also lost as a result of many other autoimmune diseases that are connected with thyroid issues include polycystic ovary syndrome and lupus erythematosus. Sometimes the use of drugs like carbimazole and propylthiouracil which are antithyroid may also lead to hair loss.

12.2 Symptoms of Thyroid-related Hair Loss

during hypothyroidism and hyperthyroidism, one may not observe the hair loss symptoms rapidly. It may also possible that one may not observe the bald spots or missed patches. Instead, the hairs may seem to get thinner overall. Each day 50 to 100 hairs fall from the head, but the good news is that this hair loss is not permanent. Thyroid controlling drugs will improve hair loss.

12.3 Treatment

The thinning of hair is may does not occur if you are suffering from mild thyroid conditions. Consulting the doctor properly will help for sure in controlling the worse conditions with the help of medication, which will not only result in thickening of the hair but may also lead to the regeneration of hair growth with time which may differ in colour or texture from the original hairs.

The medication includes levothyroxine if anyone is suffering from hypothyroidism. Propylthiouracil, methimazole, and beta-blockers will help in controlling hyperthyroidism.

Proper monitoring will be done during the medication period. In a few cases, surgery may also be required.

12.4 Natural treatments and home remedies

Some useful home remedies help to slow hair loss and regeneration of hair growth along with medicines.

❖ **Increase Iron Intake**

By increasing the iron intake, the hair loss may be controlled because ferritin levels relate to iron stores. Low levels of ferritin may lead us towards patterned hair loss.

❖ Overcome Nutritional Deficiencies

Nutritional deficiencies also contribute to hair loss. Deficiency of Vitamins B-7 and B complex, zinc, copper, iron, coenzyme Q10, vitamin C, E and A plays a major role in hair retention and loss. Hence taking multivitamins will help to increase your stores but too much intake of supplements may also lead to hair thinning.

❖ Improve Eating Habits

If you are eating a diet of whole food, it will be key for your health.

❖ Addition of anti-inflammatory foods

Adding anti-inflammatory foods like ginger and turmeric will help in improving endocrine function.

❖ Eating Herbs

Some herbs are very useful for treating hair loss that occurred from alopecia. These herbs are taken orally and include palmetto, black cohosh, dong Quai, false unicorn, chaste berry, and red clover.

❖ Applying Essentials Oils

Essential oils like arnica Montana, Cedrus atlantica, Lavandula Angustifolia, Ocimum sanctum,

Pilocarpus jabarondi, and Rosmarinus officinalis are very helpful in improving hair density.

❖ Iodine Intake check

Observe daily iodine intake as people having autoimmune thyroid disorder need to maintain the balance of iodine which otherwise may lead to many imbalances.

Kelp and other seaweeds have a high content of iodine present in them which may worsen the symptoms of hair loss.

❖ Treat hair gently

By treating the hairs gently and with care, the hair loss can be avoided i.e. don't put tight bands and use a wide-toothed comb in place of hairbrushes.

13-Thyroid Dysfunction and Weight

It has been long for a long time that a complex relationship exists between thyroid disease, metabolism, and body weight. Thyroid hormones play a significant role in the regulation of the metabolic rates in both animals and humans.

The rate of metabolism is established by measuring the amount of oxygen used by the body over a specific time. The metabolic rate at a resting state of the body is known as the basal metabolic rate (BMR). And the measurement of the BMR was one of the earliest tests that were used to determine the thyroid function of a patient. Patients with hypothyroidism had low BMRs, while individuals suffering from hyperthyroidism had high BMRs. These findings showed that low thyroid hormone levels were linked with low BMRs and high thyroid hormone levels were correlated with high BMRs.

13.1 The Link Between Hyperthyroidism and Weight Loss

Hyperthyroid individuals have an increased BMR and many patients with an overactive thyroid also suffer from some weight loss. Moreover, weight loss is directly influenced by the severity of the overactive thyroid (hyperthyroidism). For instance, if the thyroid is very overactive, the basal metabolic rate of the individual increases to an undesired level and causes an increase in the number of calories required to maintain the body weight. As higher BMR means an increase in the burning of calories. And if one does not increase the intake of calories and match it with the excess calories burned, then this will eventually result in weight loss.

As we know that our appetite is controlled by various factors and thyroid hormone levels and metabolic rate are just two components of this system. However, studies have indicated that the more severe the hyperthyroidism, the more the weight loss. Other thyroid disorders, such as in the toxic phase of thyroiditis or overuse of thyroid hormone pills can also result in weight loss. The fact that any weight loss that occurs due to hyperthyroidism is reversed or regained when the thyroid condition is treated. This shows that a direct link is present between the level of thyroid hormones, metabolism, and body weight.

13.2 Relationship between Hypothyroidism and Weight Gain

The BMR in the patient with hypothyroidism is reduced, and an underactive thyroid results in weight gain. The severe hypothyroidism the greater is the weight gain. However, the reduction in BMR due to hypothyroidism is less severe as compared to the increase seen in hyperthyroidism. This leads to less severe changes in weight due to the underactive thyroid.

The biochemistry of weight gain in hypothyroid individuals is quite complex. Research has shown that the weight gain in hypothyroid patients does not involve the accumulation of fat as in the case of conventional weight gain. Most of the extra weight that is put on by hypothyroid individuals is caused due to the accumulation of excess salt and water. But the amount of weight gain is not alarming and massive weight gain is rarely seen in hypothyroidism. And on average, depending on the severity, around 10 pounds of weight is gained as a result of hypothyroidism. Treatment of hypothyroidism can lead to weight loss, but the loss is not very prominent. As the removal of accumulated salt and water account for not more than 10% of the body weight.

Various studies have shown that thyroid hormones have been used as a tool for weight loss tool. Individuals who intend to reduce weight start taking thyroid hormones or increase the dose of already prescribed thyroid hormone to get a significant change in their weight. The excess thyroid hormone use can help in efficient weight loss as compared to that achieved through dieting, but this magic comes with a price. Excessive thyroid hormone can increase the risks of heart diseases, bone loss, muscle pain, and metabolic abnormalities.

Moreover, the weight loss caused by thyroid hormone use is temporary, and as soon as the intake of hormone is stopped, the body regains the lost weight and return to the original weight depending on the metabolic rate and appetite of the individual.

14. Other Thyroid-Related Dysfunctions

14.1 Goiter

An enlarged thyroid gland is known as a goitre. A thyroid gland is present in front of the windpipe which produces and secretes hormones that regulate growth and metabolism. Mostly the reported cases are categorized as simple goitres because they do not involve any inflammation or any detriment to thyroid function, no visible symptoms and often having no obvious cause.

The severity of the symptoms varies concerning an individual. Most of the goitres produce no prominent symptoms but when the symptoms occur a person feels tightness, cough, and hoarseness, difficulty in swallowing or in severe cases difficulty breathing with a high pitch sound.

The symptoms of an overactive thyroid can cause symptoms like nervousness, palpitations, hyperactivity, increased sweating, heat hypersensitivity, fatigue, increased appetite, loss of hair and weight loss. The symptoms of an underactive thyroid can cause symptoms like cold intolerance, constipation, forgetfulness, personality changes, hair loss, and weight gain.

14.1.1 Various Causes of Goiter

Different conditions contribute to causing a goitre.

Iodine deficiency

Iodine deficiency is considered one of the major cause of goitre around the world but this is rarely a cause in countries which a well-developed and where iodine is added to salt in daily routine.

In some parts of the world, the frequency of goitre cases is reported as high as 80% i.e. in the remote mountainous regions of southeast Asia, Latin America and central Africa. In these mentioned places the daily intake of iodine can fall below 25 micrograms (mcg) per day and the babies are often born with hypothyroidism.

To regulate metabolism, the thyroid gland requires iodine to manufacture thyroid hormones.

Autoimmune disease

The major cause of goitre in developed countries

is an autoimmune disease. Women that are over the age of 40 are at a greater risk of goitre, especially the people having a family history of this condition.

Hypothyroidism is a consequence of an underactive thyroid gland and this produces goitre. As the gland produces too little thyroid hormone, it is prompt to produce more which leads to the swelling. Usually, this is a result of Hashimoto's thyroiditis, which is a condition in which tissues of a body are attacked by the body's immune system that causes inflammation of the thyroid gland.

Hyperthyroidism is a result of an overactive thyroid gland that causes goitre. In this situation, too much thyroid hormone is produced. Usually, this is a result of Graves' disease, an autoimmune disorder in which the body's immune system turns on itself and attacks the thyroid gland which causes it to swell.

Less common causes

Some of the less common causes of goitre include

❖ **Smoking**

A chemical thiocyanate present in tobacco smoke affects the absorption of iodine in a body resulting in goitre.

- ❖ **Hormonal changes**

    Menopause, pregnancy, and puberty can affect thyroid function which results in goitre.

- ❖ **Thyroiditis**

    Inflammation that is caused by infection of bacteria or viruses can cause goitre.

- ❖ **Lithium**

    Psychiatric drugs that contain lithium can interfere with the functioning of the thyroid.

- ❖ **Overconsumption of iodine**

    If iodine is consumed in a large amount, then too much iodine can also cause goitre.

- ❖ **Radiation therapy**

    This can activate a swollen thyroid, especially when administered to the neck.

14.1.2 Diagnosis of Goiter

Goitre can only be diagnosed with a physical examination of the neck, feeling for a swelling. To check for goitre, the doctor may ask the patient to swallow. Once the doctor diagnoses a patient for goitre, the underlying problems with the thyroid function should be evaluated and the patient should be screened for hyperthyroidism or hypothyroidism.

TSH and T4 levels are measured in the blood to test thyroid function. A cautiously controlled feedback mechanism means that TSH encourages the thyroid for the production of excess thyroxine than it is required while T4 tells the thyroid to stop producing extra thyroxine.

In an overactive thyroid, TSH levels are found to be low or non-existent while T4 levels are high. People having an underactive thyroid, the reverse is true. TSH levels are high and T4 levels are low. Triiodothyronine is another hormone that is measured in some cases of an overactive gland, such as suspected Graves' disease.

In few cases of goitre, specialist tests may be arranged, i.e. Radioactive iodine scan in which a comprehensive picture of the gland is provided, followed by an injection of radioactive iodine. Ultrasound Scan evaluates the gland and size of the goitre and Fine-Needle Aspiration is a type of biopsy is done to take a sample of the cells from the gland if cancer is suspected.

The goitres that are caused by overactive thyroid or hyperthyroidism, the treatment focus to counter the production of an excess hormone. For this purpose, anti-thyroid drugs, such as ethionamide drugs are given to reduce the excessive hormone levels gradually.

Radioactive iodine is also a treatment to decrease thyroid function and to stop hormone production that causes hyperthyroidism.

The goitres that are caused by underactive thyroid or hypothyroidism, a treatment is a synthetic replacement of thyroid hormone. The dosage of synthetic thyroxine T4 is increased gradually until the body restores the normal thyroid levels.

14.1.3 Goiter Surgery

The goitre surgery is required in such critical cases where goitre is causing some problems in swallowing and difficulty in breathing. This surgery is done under general anaesthesia to remove part of the thyroid gland.

14.1.4 Best Diet for Goiter

Iodine is not present in a good amount in plants, and vegetarian food may lack enough iodine. Dietary iodine is found in seafood (salmon, tuna, halibut, shrimp, etc.), plants that are grown in iodine-rich soil, cow's milk, and eggs (good iodine and selenium are present in the yolk).

Mostly the simple type of goitres can be prevented by taking a proper amount of iodine, which is added to table salt in many countries. A wide range of iodine supplements is also available online. In cases where symptoms are visible, active treatment of goitre is done. But if the goitre is small and thyroid is functioning normally, treatment is mostly not offered.

14.2 Thyroid Nodules

Nodules are termed as "solid or lump having fluid" within the thyroid gland. This may vary in size and location. The majority of the nodules do not cause any symptoms and can only be identified during a manual examination of the thyroid gland or by doing an ultrasound of a thyroid.

Large-sized nodules may result in a visible swelling of the thyroid or neck. These nodules may cause pain, difficulty in swallowing and breathing. There are also types of nodules that produce thyroid hormones which result in hyperthyroidism.

Around 50% of adults in America are diagnosed with thyroid nodules. Women suffer three times more than men. About 30% of women when they reach the age of 30s are diagnosed with at least one while most of the women develop a thyroid at the age of 50s.

14.2.1 Symptoms of Nodules

The symptoms of thyroid nodules are not much observable. One can only notice them in a form of lump appearing on the neck or a doctor might locate these nodules during a physical exam or when a CT scans or imaging tests like ultrasounds are done for any other reasons.

Luckily, most of the nodules show symptoms but these symptoms can be manifested rarely i.e. a suffered person may feel pain in neck, ear or jaw. One can also feel a problem while breathing, swallowing or a tickle in the throat if the nodule is large. Hoarseness if the nodules affect the nerve that controls the vocal cords. This can also be related to thyroid cancer. The excessive amount of thyroxine production generates a symptom of hyperthyroidism that includes tremors, nervousness, unexplained weight loss, and erratic heartbeat.

If the thyroid test results of a person are not in a normal range than a person should get himself examined for nodules.

14.2.2 Causes of Nodules Formation

People suffering from Hashimoto have nodules which are considered as the root causes of thyroid nodules. Some other causes of thyroid nodules are given below:

❖ Chronic Inflammation of the thyroid

A chronic inflammation that is linked with autoimmune thyroid conditions may increase the risk for thyroid nodules and hence the inflammation connected with autoimmune thyroiditis can further enlarge nodules. With Hashimoto's, the body creates such antibodies that normal proteins produced by the thyroid gland which in turn results in the development of malignant nodules that might be cancerous. This thyroid might also form pseudo-nodules that may come and go.

❖ Nutritional deficiencies

Various nutritional deficiencies caused by lack of proper diet can result in the insufficiency of iodine, selenium and Vitamin D in the body. The deficiency of iodine in a body typically results in a multinodular goitre but with Hashimoto's, the excess in iodine is far more likely to cause nodules. A deficiency in selenium is also a potential cause of nodules and supplements use can improve thyroid and small size modules. Adding fish, nuts, yoghurt, and fruits to our diet can improve the severity of thyroid nodules.

❖ Toxins

Various toxins that enter our body from the

environment and food can negatively affect the thyroid and most of the time this cause of nodules is overlooked. People living near petrochemical industry areas are exposed to radiation exposure like Chernobyl and nickel toxicity, greatly contributes to the development of nodules in individuals who suffer from Hashimoto's disease.

❖ Pregnancy and Hormonal changes

Most of the time, women develop thyroid nodules during pregnancy. But the cause of nodules during pregnancy is still not much clear and many studies suggest that this may be due to negative iodine balance linked with pregnancy.

❖ H.Pylori Infections

H. Pylori infections are considered as a trigger of Hashimoto's and a study shows that a person suffering from Hashimoto's in one Iranian has been found in almost 50% of patients. According to a theory of molecular mimicry, the thyroid gland is attacked by its immune system when it gets infected with any pathogenic organism. Such an infection increases the autoimmune attack on the thyroid that results in the production of a thyroid nodule.

❖ Food and Diet

Food sensitivities are also one of the reason of

nodules as some food attack on thyroid and increase the level of chronic inflammation. Moreover, an imbalance in blood sugars may also contribute to a greater risk of thyroid nodules. Overuse of fast food and processed meals can increase the risk of developing thyroid nodules.

❖ **Treatment**

Most doctors recommend physical monitoring through regular checkups. Thyroid hormone suppression therapy can lower the production of TSH and decrease the growth of thyroid tissues. Surgery may also be recommended if the benign nodule is large and creates difficulty in breathing or swallowing.

14.2.3 Diet and Lifestyle Changes to Reduce Nodules

Changes in diet and lifestyle patterns contribute a lot to reduce thyroid nodules. Some tips are discussed below:

❖ **Add nutrients like Iodine, Selenium and Vitamin D in the diet**

People having low iodine levels may get benefit by taking multivitamins with iodine like Nutrient 950 from Pure Encapsulations. People suffering from Hashimoto's need a dose of up to 250mcg of iodine per day which is found to be helpful. However, the dose above 300mcg can be inflammatory. Taking Vitamin D and Selenium supplements may also help in the reduction of thyroid nodules.

❖ **Remove toxins from a body**

By supporting the liver detoxification methods for opting non-toxic, natural personal products can help a lot to reduce the body's toxic burden and improving optimal thyroid health. Various fruits and vegetables, including avocadoes, apples, citrus, asparagus, green leafy vegetables, beetroot and, carrot are excellent detox agents and can be used to remove unwanted toxins from the body protect the thyroid and other parts of the body.

❖ **Address underlying infections**

Infections like *H. Pylori* and *Blastocystis hominis* are considered as a root cause and activate Hashimoto's and develop thyroid nodules. By addressing such infections one can eliminate thyroid nodules as well as the risk of an autoimmune attack on the thyroid. Taking vitamin E supplements and omega 3 oils can help improve the immune system and can aid in removing any underlying infections.

❖ **Alter diet plan and remove food sensitivities**

By balancing blood sugar will help a lot in shrinking thyroid nodules. Also, eliminating common food sensitivities like gluten and dairy can help in reducing the size of nodules.

❖ **Add smart supplements**

Some studies show that the elimination of nodules is possible by consuming the systemic enzyme Wobenzym and other with turmeric. Turmeric is a powerful anti-inflammatory spice and can help reduce inflammation in the thyroid gland.

❖ **Address estrogen dominance**

Excess amounts of estrogen in a body activate the thyroid nodules. Estrogen levels may increase during pregnancy or by using birth control pills, but it rebalances on its own after delivery or stops using pills. but if estrogen levels do not rebalance even after delivery or stopped using pills than one must consider other reasons like food alteration, supplements, and progesterone to balance the hormones.

❖ **Give thought to Echo therapy (HIFU ablation)**

Studies suggest that a single sitting of high-intensity focused ultrasound (HIFU) ablation may be more beneficial than thyroidectomy. In one study it is observed that the patients who underwent HIFU ablation did not scar had a limited hospital stay and were less likely to have voice pitch problems after a month of treatment. But this method is only available currently in a few clinics in Europe.

15. Role of Microbiota in Thyroid Diseases

The community of bacteria living in our gut, termed as the gut microbiota, has a significant effect on the health and wellbeing of the body. Various diseases and metabolic disorders have also been identified to have a link with the microbiota of the affected individual. Researches have shown that an altered composition of microbiota significantly affects the thyroid function and increases the incidence of thyroid disorders, including Graves's diseases (GD) and Hashimoto's thyroiditis (HT).

Microbes affect the level of thyroid hormone in the body. They do so by interfering with different metabolic processes such as regulation of uptake of iodine uptake, its degradation, and enterohepatic cycling. Moreover, various minerals that are present in our diet interact with the microbes and influence their interaction with the host. Examples of such minerals include zinc, iron, and selenium.

There is a definite influence of minerals on interactions between host and microbiota, particularly selenium, iron, and zinc. Microbiota may also affect the uptake of L-thyroxine and influence the action of propylthiouracil (PTU), which can directly affect the function of the thyroid gland. It is now known that thyroid disorders are associated with the type of microbiota present in the gut.

15.1 Link between Thyroid Hormones and Microbiota

As we know that the primary functions of the thyroid gland include uptake of iodine uptake, hormone recycling, and uptake and metabolism of the drug. The microbiota of the individual can affect the thyroid function at different levels.

The microbiota has been reported to affect the incidence of AID, regulate the levels of estrogen and iodine, and obesity. It influences the metabolism of the anti-hyperthyroid drug propylthiouracil (PTU), regulates the enterohepatic cycling of thyroid hormones, and affects the bioavailability of levothyroxine (L-thyroxine), that is essential to produce thyroid hormone.

Further, various host factors including diet (iodine intake), region, age, obesity, sex hormones, and AID also determine the composition of the intestinal microbiota.

In this way, a reciprocate relationship exists between thyroid hormone and microbiota (Figure 6). In this relationship various events can occur, which are given below:

- Iodine can have toxic effects on the microbiota, and the microbiota that influences the uptake of iodine
- Autoimmune thyroid disease (AITD) patients have an altered population of their microbiota. While leaky gut syndrome (LGS) is induced by the overgrowth of bacteria and can increase the prevalence of AITD. So, they are interrelated
- Estrogen hormone recycling is carried out by microbiota and the composition of the microbiota is distinct in women and men.
- Obesity can cause changes in microbiota, and faecal transfer can affect the phenotype and change it from obese to slim.

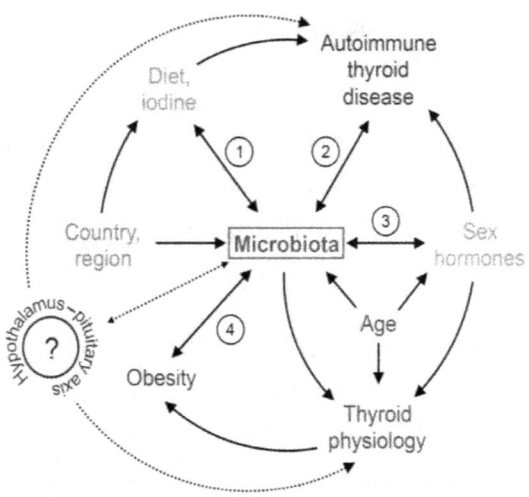

Figure 6. The interrelationship between gut microbiota and thyroid hormones

Various effects of the microbiota on the function of the thyroid gland, related disorders and the proposed treatments using microbes are described in the next section.

15.2 Gut Microbiome and Thyroid Disorder

The microbiota of the intestine has been known to play a major role in the body. It maintains the homeostasis of the gastrointestinal tract and has been identified as a key mediator of disorders. Gut microbiota has also been linked with various other problems, such as heart diseases, depression, obesity, neurodegenerative diseases, diabetes, inflammatory bowel disorder, immunological disorders, and cancer.

The role of microbiota explains the reason why the high prevalence of goitre in South India is not correlated with low iodine intake and in Japan where hypothyroidism is more prevalent in iodine-rich areas as compared to its prevalence in iodine-poor areas. The microbes inhabiting the gut have the ability to interfere with the metabolism of iodine and can affect the function of the thyroid gland and cause other metabolic problems.

Diabetes mellitus is considered as the most common pathology of the endocrine system, followed by thyroid dysfunctions. The thyroid disorders are caused by various underlying factors and there are various other risk factors associated with them, which include genetic disposition, iodine deficiency, sex, and age. The level of thyroid-stimulating hormone (TSH) increases with age, but thyroid disorders are most common in the middle-aged population [8]. Autoimmune diseases (AIDs) of the thyroid gland are more common in women than in men.

15.3 Role of the Gut Microbiota in Autoimmune Thyroid Diseases

The incidence of autoimmune thyroid disease is very high and is considered the most common organ-specific autoimmune disease in the world. The role of gut microbiota is very powerful in triggering the autoimmune against the thyroid gland. Various metabolic products of the microorganism, such as short-chain fatty acids (SCFAs) act as an energy source for the cells of the intestine. And these SCFAs together with thyroid hormones carry out the differentiation and binding of the enterocytes. This is the positive role that gut microbiota plays in the body.

In an abnormal microbial community, various mechanisms such as the production of self-antigens by modifications of proteins, induction of T helper cells and activation of Toll-like receptors by the lipopolysaccharides of the microbial cell wall can lead to loss of integrity of enterocytes. This results in a condition called leaky gut and can elicit various immune responses in the body. These altered responses promote the development of AID and can lead to Graves' disease and Hashimoto's disease. These two autoimmune-based thyroid disorders, GD and HD, have different immunological mechanisms.

The primary immunologic features of Graves' disease involve the presence of circulating antibodies against the TSH receptor. Hashimotos's disease involves the presence of antibodies against thyroglobulin and thyroid-peroxidase that attack the thyroid gland and causes the destruction of thyroid tissues. HD is also marked by the presence of autoreactive T cells. The role of gut microbiota in the manifestation and mechanism of the two diseases can be also different.

As the severity of these autoimmune thyroid diseases is not proportional to the level of antibodies in the blood. Moreover, other symptoms of GD such as depression and anxiety don't have a direct link with thyroid autoimmunity or thyroid function. And it is postulated that the gut microbiome mediates the behavioural effects of thyroid disorder. It has been reported that the higher level of *Enterobacteriaceae* and *Actinobacteria* in the gut are linked with the manifestation of mood disorder in thyroid patient as compared to normal individuals.

Other species of bacteria, including *Lactobacillaceae* and *Bifidobacteria* are decreased and *Clostridium* population was increased in individuals with thyroid dysfunction and have behavioural problems. These bacteria have been known to produce gamma-aminobutyric acid (GABA) and its low level are linked with depression and anxiety.

As we know that metabolic products of microbes can affect the central nervous system (CNS) and can cause various changes. A change in microbiota from conventional to specific in rats resulted in an increased incidence of Hashimotos's disease. As *Lactobacillus spp.* and *Bifidobacterium spp.* may result in the induction of immune response and production of antibodies that cross-react with thyroid peroxidase and thyroglobulin.

Gut microbiota composition also plays an important role in increasing the vulnerability of mouse strains to Graves' disease. Various bacterial genera, including *Allobaculum, Ureaplasma*, and *Limibacter* have been linked with the presence of GD. Moreover, a high prevalence of *Prevotellaceae,* and lower abundance of *Enterobacteriaceae*, and *Veillonellaceae* were found in disease group compared to normal. And patients with hyperthyroidism had more abundance of *Enterococcus spp.,* and decreased population of *Lactobacillaceae*. Individuals with autoimmune-thyroid disorder produce three different types of antibodies, which include anti-gliadin, anti-yeast (*Saccharomyces cerevisiae*) and anti-transglutaminase antibodies.

15.4 Role of Microbiota in Therapy of Thyroid Disorders

The effectiveness of oral L-thyroxine supplementation by its absorption in the gastrointestinal tract by different transporters is dependent on the efficiency of gut microbes to breakdown and oxidize the thyroid hormones. A higher amount of microbiota requires higher doses of L-thyroxine. Small intestinal bacterial overgrowth (SIBO) is a condition characterized by the presence of an overgrowth of microorganisms and a CFU (colony forming unit) of more than 106 CFU in an intestinal sample.

Hypothyroidism leads to an increase in stomach pH and decrease in the gastric motility which can contribute greatly to bacterial growth. Hypothyroid patients suffer from reduced degradation of protein in the gut, thus providing ideal environment for the bacteria to grow exponentially. Research showed that altered colonization of the gastrointestinal tract with microbes such as due to *Helicobacter pylori* infections can lead to increased dosage requirement of L-thyroxine. That means individuals with H. pylori infection lead to increased pH of the gut and increased pH can lead to dissolution of L-thyroxine, and decreased absorption.

Research has shown that the intestinal microbiota influences the metabolism and absorption of around 30 different drugs. That is why the use of L-thyroxine for the treatment of hyperthyroidism can be affected by the gut microbiota. Moreover, the bile acids released by the microbes of the gut can influence the function of cytochrome P450 present in the liver cells.

15.5 Role of the Gut Microbiota in Metabolism of Thyroid Hormone

High dose of iodine can prove to be toxic for the gut microbiota. This toxicity is caused by binding of iodine to the amino acids present on the bacterial cell membrane and by oxidation of membrane components and cytoplasmic organelles. Various other minerals such as zinc, selenium and iron support the function and health of the thyroid gland. The thyroid gland has the highest amount of selenium in the body. And is required by many enzymes involved in the thyroid metabolism. These enzymes include glutathione peroxidase, type I, II, and III iodothyronine deiodinases and thioredoxin reductase. Thyroperoxidase has iron in the active centre and zinc improves the activity of D2 which converts inactive T4 to active T3.

Research shows that dysfunction of is associated with abnormal levels of iron, zinc, selenium and other essential minerals. Zinc deficiency leads to a decreased level of thyroid hormones, TSH, T4, and T3, in the serum. It is known that a reciprocal relationship exists between zinc and thyroid metabolism as hypothyroidism leads to zinc deficiency and lack of zinc intake through diet and supplements can lead to hypothyroidism.

Selenium, zinc iron and other minerals can also influence the t microbial flora of the gut. The bacteria in the microbial community compete for minerals with the host, for instance for selenium as they also need it for their growth and metabolism. Resident microbes can degrade the selenium and renders it unavailable for the host. Selenium has been reported to increase the microbial diversity in mice and promotes the growth of Bifidobacterium adolescentis in the gut.

Iron is absorbed best at lower pH and microbes play important role in absorption by producing fatty acids and decreasing the pH in the colon. as Fe. Bacteria also possess high-affinity proteins for iron, called the siderophores, that facilitate the uptake of iron. Such siderophores are expressed in high quantity in pathogenic bacterial strains. Deficiency of iron in the diet can limit the bacterial growth, while an iron-rich diet decreases the microbial diversity. Use of iron supplementation in humans has been linked with an increased population of Enterobacteriaceae and decreased Lactobacillaceae members. This results due to the action of inflammation in stimulating the microbiome and was accompanied by increased production of formate and lactate.

The relationship between the gastrointestinal tract and the thyroid gland has been known since last century and is known as hypogastric syndrome, also called the autoimmune metaplastic atrophic gastritis (AMAG). The correlation of both diseases is explained by the fact that both have a common embryonic origin. The origin of thyroid follicular cells and gastric mucosal cells is same as the thyroid gland develops from primitive gut cells. Moreover, they both can take up iodine and express similar enzyme, peroxidase. and they express similar peroxidases (gastric peroxidase and thyroperoxidase). A certain microbiota composition has been linked with increasing the risk of both diseases in various individuals. For instance, the reduction of Lactobacillaceae and Bifidobacteriaceae have been linked with an increased incidence of thyroid diseases.

Gut microbiota is very important in the regulation of thyroid function as about 20% the conversion of T4 to T3 takes place in the GI tract by intestinal sulfates. Bile acids also present an interesting link between gut bacteria and thyroid function. Primary bile acids that are secreted by the gallbladder into the small intestine are metabolized by the gut bacteria and converted into secondary bile acids. These secondary bile acids boost the activity of iodothyronine that converts T4 into T3. In this way, the function and wellbeing of gut microbiota and thyroid gland are interconnected. It is now known that by improving the gut microflora can have positive effects on the thyroid function. There are various researches that highlight the importance of a healthy diet, rich in fibres and good bacteria, for the improvement of gut microbiota. Use of probiotic supplements has become popular in treating gastrointestinal disorders and thyroid dysfunction.

In the next section we will discuss the foods and diet plan for acquiring a healthy gut microbiota that can significantly improve the symptoms of thyroid dysfunction.

15.6 Healing the Gut to Improve Thyroid Function

Diet can be used as the best medicine if taken

with wisdom. Thyroid problems are the most common disorders that can be improved by healthy eating and adding beneficial foods to our diet. The role of gut microbiome in improving the thyroid functions have helped us to formulate microbiome-improving diet routine, that is given below

15.6.1 Increased Intake of Fermentable Fiber

As described before the metabolic products of bacteria act as a strong modulators of the endocrine system. That is why it is advised that we consume fermentable fibres such as sweet potato, cassava, and plantains (belong to banana family) in our diet. Such a diet will allow the gut bacteria to ferment the fibres and produce short-chain fatty acids (SCFAs). These fatty acids regulate gene expression and have epigenetic effects. They have been found to regulate the expression of thyroid receptor gene in humans. Among other important functions, these are responsible for decreasing the pH in the gut which aids in the conversion of thyroid hormone from its inactive to an active form.

15.6.2 Use of Probiotics

The improvement of gut microflora using probiotic supplements have been recommended to improve the symptoms of thyroid disorders. in Reports have shown that the addition of lactic acid bacteria to broiler chickens is linked with an increase in thyroid hormones in the body. Similarly, the use of *Lactobacillus reuteri* supplementation proved to be beneficial for thyroid function in rats. Various fermented vegetables, including kimchi and sauerkraut are considered as useful probiotics as they are a good source of lactic acid-producing bacteria. Other examples of good probiotics that have been recommended for improving gut and thyroid function include Fermented dairy products such as kefir and yoghurt.

15.6.3 Keeping a Check on SIBO or Other Gut Pathogens

People with thyroid problems are advised to get themselves checked for overgrowth of microorganisms in the gut. As hypothyroidism can affect the gastric mobility, which can lead to increased risk of microbial overgrowth (SIBO). Bacterial overgrowth can cause abdominal discomfort, increased bloating, and can even cause typhoid. So, it is recommended that people with thyroid issues get their gut checked for SIBO and manage the population of their gut microbiome.

15.6.4 Practice Gut-Friendly Regime

Our gut is the centre of all the functions of the body, and it gets little time to rest and heal. So, it is recommended that we eat such food that is gut-friendly and does not burden the gastric tract. Further, it is necessary that we adopt a healthy lifestyle, which includes exercise and meditation. People with thyroid issues or at risk of developing thyroid problems should remove pro-inflammatory food from their diets, such as processed food, fast food and bakery products. It is advised that we increase the intake of gut-healing foods such as bone broth and fibres. It is also important to learn to manage our stresses as they can negatively affect our gut and appetite. Research has shown that by healing the gut greatly helps in managing the symptoms of thyroid disorder.

16. Hashimoto's Protocol and Diet Plan for Thyroid

Hashimoto's Protocol provides a practical track at the root of the disease for healing and reversing the autoimmune damage. The first step includes an active start two-week detox program that incorporates foods to eat and to avoid inflammatory foods, advice to take supplements to support the liver, and an adrenal recovery plan. One can also create a personalized plan which involves foods, supplements, and other lifestyle interventions according to their body's own exclusive Hashimoto's triggers. One should try to understand ancient idioms which say, "Let food be your medicine" and "All diseases start in the gut".

16.1 Thyroid Diet plan

Diet includes a vast meaning. Sometimes diet is when a person wants to lose weight but often diet is taken as a nourishing food change that brings joy and relief. But in general, diet is a protocol, a way of living and eating that can free a person from all the fatigue, depression, extra weight, anxiety, frustrations, and infertility.

Every person has its own opinion. Some people believe that there is no scientific evidence that links to food that improves thyroid problems. Even if there is no scientific evidence that food is related to thyroid healing even than there is no harm in trying something new and different for three weeks and just check how it feels.

It is very well known that 90% of the hypo-and hyperthyroidism results from an autoimmune disorder. Most of the hypothyroid conditions are Hashimoto's and most hyperthyroid conditions are Graves' disease, which clearly tells that an immune system is attacked by a thyroid. Since an immune system resides in the gut or intestine, so one should consider rebuilding its digestive system.

16.2 Three Pillars of Diet Plan

Before heading towards a thyroid diet plan, let's check out the three pillars of the diet plan.

Number 1: what should a person REMOVE from his current diet and lifestyle that is damaging his immune system and thyroid?

Number 2: what should a person ADD to his life

to boost his immune system, detox his body, and help to improve his thyroid?

Number 3: how do a person creates a BALANCE in his eating habits and lifestyle?

Here are the answers to the above three questions.

16.2.1 Pillar 1: Remove what is damaging and toxic for a thyroid

a) Sugar fluctuations

This is very important in a thyroid diet plan to normalize sugar cravings, hypoglycemia or insulin resistance. Without fixing sugar issues, the thyroid will never get improved. This happens because the pancreas is accountable for sugar metabolism. Same as thyroid, the pancreas is a part of the endocrine system. So, it can be clearly observed that these glands are all intricately interconnected. To control a diet for thyroid health, here are few tips are given below:

During product purchasing, start reading the products' labels to check how much sugar is present in that food; 4g = 1 teaspoon. For example, a Frappuccino will have 64g of sugar which means it contains 16 spoons of sugar. Activia's yoghurt which is claimed as healthy food contains 7 spoons of sugar. But if a person is having a sugar problem then he should not consume more than 5 spoons of sugar per day.

It is recommended that we begin the day with a high-protein and a goof fat breakfast. This is considered as a big secret in an industry of weight loss. This will help the person to stabilize his sugar level for the whole day. A person will not crash at 11 am and surely will not crave sugar and snacks during the day.

One should reduce the use of processed carbs. As a carbs obsessed nation, carbs add up about 50-60% of most people's diet, much of which is coming from grains. Grains carry starch that helps to feed the pathogenic bacteria in a gut and aggravate the problem.

Also reduce starch because again the sugar content is present in it especially from potatoes, sweet potatoes, and processed food.

b) Food intolerances

Today, gluten-free and dairy-free products are available at all health stores. This is happening because people are trying to get off gluten, dairy, corn, and eggs and are experiencing a significant change. But these eliminations from the diet have produced clear and unbiased results. If a person gets a food intolerance test done, they will be far from accuracy. Gluten is not a much famous food for contributing to thyroid conditions and eliminating it is key. However, often one should need to cut out more than just gluten if he is wishing to shape up his diet regarding thyroid fitness.

c) Fixing the Gut

It is already mentioned above that most thyroid conditions are auto-immune diseases. Gut consists of tons of lymphocytes and many other immune cells that protect the body from different viruses, bacteria, and other attackers. This is considered as the main reason why most of the people having thyroid conditions suffer from different problems like constipation, bloating, gas or diarrhoea. A change in diet plan helps the gut enormously as it a very famous idiom that "All disease begins in the gut".

d) Reduce toxicity

A person should reduce the toxins he ingests from different additives, preservatives, artificial sweeteners, excessive sodium, and trans-fats. One should try his best to eliminate all the toxins hiding in houses. Toxicity of water is a major problem considered in thyroid conditions. The US has started adding fluoride in public water systems which is now helping out in slow down the thyroid. It is believed that fluoride leach on to thyroid cells, inhibits the uptake of iodine and hence the production of thyroid hormone is altered.

e) Reduce stress and adrenal fatigue

This point mainly relates to women, but men can suffer from endocrine stress in older age. It is not possible to fix a thyroid without fixing the adrenals. The adrenals are a part of the endocrine system and boost up when a person is stressed out. One should look up the adrenal fatigue symptoms in his life and must de-stressed them by consulting with a therapist or life coach, take a proper medication if required and always think positively will work as a key. Another reason for stress is caused by chronic digestive issues. Whenever the small or large intestine feels distressed, the body will automatically feel itself in a state of stress.

Pillar 2: Add food to boost the immune system, detox and improving thyroid

a) Soy

The research suggested that phytoestrogens that are present in soybeans and foods that are rich in soy discourage the activity of an enzyme that creates thyroid hormones.

b) Iodine-rich food

Sometimes hypothyroidism is caused by a deficiency of sufficient iodine. So, in such cases, using the food that is rich in iodized salt or iodine-rich foods can be beneficial. One can also take supplements after consulting a doctor.

c) Iron and calcium supplements

By taking iron and calcium supplements can also help in improving the effectiveness of thyroid medications.

d) High-fibre foods

Usually, high fibre food is advised but it should be taken two hours before or after taking thyroid medicine because it may interfere with the absorption of the medicine.

e) Antioxidants

Antioxidant food like blueberries, tomatoes, bell peppers, and other foods that help in detox can help in improving the health and thyroid gland. Taking food that is rich in vitamin B i.e. whole grains is also advised.

f) Proteins and fats

Proteins and fats are considered as a building block of a digestive tract and hormones. Asian and

Europeans who consumes fat-rich diets enjoy far better health than Americans who consume a low-fat diet. Food with good fat includes avocados, walnuts, coconut oil, and coconut butter. Animal fat is also considered the best in restoring problematic digestion. Animals fat includes clarified butter, simple butter, chicken and beef fat.

16.2.3 Pillar 3: Create a balance in eating and lifestyle

Try eating a balanced diet that gives a body all the essential nutrients it requires to function properly. Do not eat too much in one go or don't eat too little as well. Try eating in at least five small portions of a variety of food and vegetables every day.

A person's daily lifestyle is also very important. If a person plays any sports, do dancing or yoga, it is very essential to engage himself in such a limit that does not drain his adrenals or thyroids. One's lifestyle should give him a sense of joy and comfort rather than fatigue. In short, do not do excessive cardio or workouts as well and switch to light weightlifting, yoga, gentle cycling, hiking, etc.

16.3 Recommended Meal Plan for Hypothyroid Individual

This meal plan is for hypothyroidism and weight loss. This is a dietitian made plan that will help to make life easier and more joyful while learning that what one should and should not eat with an underactive thyroid.

Day 1

- **Breakfast:** Take one large banana.
- **Lunch:** Eat Greek Yogurt Tuna salad. Greek yoghurt contains high protein and low sugar levels. However, this tuna is a rich source of iodine and healthy omega-3 fats.
- **Snack:** Take 2-3 Brazil nuts because they contain high protein, fibre, and healthy fats. Brazil nuts are also an excellent source of selenium that is good for thyroid health. They also do not participate in increasing body weight.

Day 2

- **Breakfast:** Prepare an overnight chocolate chia pudding. Chia seeds are a great source of magnesium, protein, and fibre.
- **Lunch:** Eat a gluten-free sandwich with tinned tuna with topping.

- **Dinner:** Make egg shakshuka plus rice. This Tunisian dish is a great source of vegetables and eggs with a good source of iodine as well and rice is naturally gluten-free.
- **Snack:** Prepare one cup of carrot and cucumber sticks with cottage cheese or hummus i.e. DIY spicy peanut Butter Hummus.

Day 3

- **Breakfast:** Eat gluten-free toast with eggs.
- **Lunch:** Prepare Middle-Eastern mason jar salad. This is such a simple dish. Mason jar is optional, but one will need a jar of some type.
- **Dinner:** Take eating shrimps, zucchini and pesto angel pasta. Always use gluten-free pasta for making this dinner. Shrimps are also a good source of iodine.

Day 4

- **Snack:** Eat one banana as a starter.
- **Breakfast:** Make a green monster smoothie. This will require a blender, and this is also another way of making use of chia seeds and adding them to your diet.
- **Lunch:** Prepare pumpkin soup. They help in lowering the calorie than regular meals, rich

in vegetables and keep a person feel full for longer.
- **Dinner:** Just eat leftovers at dinner.
- **Snack:** Only take 2-3 Brazil nuts.

Day 5

- **Breakfast:** One can eat his favourite dish.
- **Lunch:** Eat leftover or a person may eat what he likes at that time.
- **Dinner:** Eat one pot cheesy taco skillet.
- **Snack:** Prepare 1 cup of carrot and cucumber sticks plus cottage cheese or hummus.

Day 6

- **Breakfast:** One can eat his favourite dish.
- **Lunch:** Quinoa salad with nuts. Quinoa is a variable grain that contains high protein and is gluten-free.
- **Dinner:** One can eat his favourite dish, to go for leftovers or to eat out is his choice.

Day 7

- **Breakfast:** Start the day by eating California sweet potato hash with feta and eggs. Eating sweet potatoes in the morning is beneficial too.
- **Lunch:** Again, one can eat his favourite dish.

- **Dinner:** Prepare crusted chicken parmesan with vegetables at dinner. This is a wonderful and delicious way of serving chicken.
- **Snack:** Eat about 200g of plain Greek yoghurt with one small banana.

16.4 Things to consider before adopting any diet plan

One should consult a doctor or dietitian first before considering an alteration in his diet or fitness regime. Goitrogens and soy are only beneficial if consumed in moderate amounts. Moreover, if legumes give a person digestive discomfort, he should stop using it. This diet plan does not tell us about the consumption of water or drinks, but one should keep himself hydrated all the time. Taking tea is also a good choice but more than 300mg per day of caffeine is not good for the thyroid.

17. Treatment of Thyroid via Detox

Various environmental factors, including exposure to radiation and toxins, can have adverse effects on thyroid function. There are many toxins that can disrupt the homeostasis of the thyroid gland and can trigger an immune response against the thyroid tissue. This autoimmune response leads to Hashimotos's thyroiditis can researches now suggest that by removing harmful toxins from our body, we can considerably decrease the risk of developing thyroid and other dysfunctions in the body. Detoxing our body is the need of time as it is almost impossible to protect ourselves from the ubiquitously spread toxins in the environment. There are various detox regimes can have proved to be effective in aiding the liver functions and in removing toxins our body.

Liver carries out the process of degradation and removal of unwanted chemicals and toxins from the body. There are three potent habits that can help you detox your body; they are described below:

❖ Move the Muscles

Adopting a healthy lifestyle and making exercise a permanent part of your daily regime is very helpful for the health of thyroid. Individuals with decreased activity of the thyroid gland can improve their symptoms by doing high-intensity training and workouts, such as running, swimming and cycling. Such exercises increase the sensitivity of the body tissues to the thyroid hormone and promote the production of thyroid hormone by the thyroid gland.

It is a fact that hypothyroidism lessens the capacity and urge to exercise capacity but hormone replacement therapy by using thyroxine, the capacity to exercise and remain physically active can be attained back. Use of hormone replacement along with regular physical exercise has shown improvement in the thyroid function and increase the physical and mental and status of the hypothyroid patient. That is why it is highly recommended that every young to middle-aged patient with hypothyroidism should do regular physical exercise to cope with their symptoms and enjoy a better life.

Research has proven that doing gentle exercise yoga and walking, can also stimulate thyroid gland secretion and improves tissue sensitivity to the thyroid hormone. The metabolism of thyroid hormone in the body is also altered due to various physiological changes, which can change the deiodination pathway and lead to a change in the serum thyroid levels. The biological effects of short-term changes in the thyroid hormones are important in the adjustment of the body to stressful states. A link has been recognized through studies that by a training routine of 80 km/week helps improve the level of thyroid hormones in the body. But regardless of the level of your fitness, it is established that increasing physical activity can help boost your thyroid function.

❖ Burn the Fat

Another effective way of detoxing your body is by spending time in a sauna or steam room. It is characterized as a great way to relax and help flush thyroid-damaging toxins out of the body. The heat causes sweating that removes the toxins out of the system that can be harmful to the body. Further, regular visits to sauna and steam rooms can aid with weight loss, which can help manage the symptoms of thyroid dysfunction. Burning and loss of fat leads to the removal of toxins like pesticides and PCBs that reside in the fat cells. It is recommended that thyroid patients should be more involved in fat burning activities that help them detox and feel healthier.

- ❖ **Eat More Fiber**

The best detox starts in the gut. It is recommended that we eat a high-fiber diet. This can be achieved by adding fruits, vegetables, seeds, nuts, other plant-based foods in our diet. This will help us in boosting our health, enhance the immune system, and reduce the level of toxins in the body. A fiber-rich diet helps to improve the detoxing function of the kidney and liver, as they bind the toxins and move them out of the body without causing any burden on other organs. It is advised that we take different sources of fiber as different variety of fiber have different benefits for the body.

Everyone has a different metabolic rate and the burden of toxins for everyone is also different. We can adopt different measures to boost the natural detox system and that is the best thing we can do to remove toxins from our system. A detox diet does not do anything that a body can't do and only optimizes the body's natural detoxification system. Detox diets are tempting and once you develop the taste it helps the body to handle toxins and other unwanted substances.

❖ Consumes plenty of water

The only function of water is not only to quench one's thirst, but it does so much for a body. It regulates the body's temperature, helps in the digestion process, lubricates joints and helps absorb nutrients. It also plays a major role in detoxifying by removing waste products from a body.

The cells of a body continuously repair itself to function properly and break down all the nutrients present in a body to use as energy. However, all the processes take place inside a body release wastes i.e. in a form of urea and carbon dioxide, but if they are allowed to stay in the body, they will start causing harm.

Water helps in transporting the waste produced in a body efficiently by removing through the urination process, breathing or sweating. Hence, staying properly hydrated is very important for detoxification.

A requirement of water is different for men and women. An appropriate daily intake of water is 125 ounces (3.7 liters) for men and 91 ounces (2.7 liters) for women. But this amount can vary depending upon a person's activity level, where a person lives and what he eats.

❖ Reduce sugar and processed foods intake

Presently, sugar and processed food are the root cause of destroying public health. Consumption of high sugar and processed food is a root cause of obesity and other chronic diseases such as heart disease, cancer, and diabetes.

These diseases slow down the body's ability to naturally detoxify itself by harming the organs that play an important role i.e. liver and kidneys. Consumption of highly sugary products can cause fatty liver which alters the functions of a liver.

Hence, one should try to eat healthy food like fruits and vegetables instead of junk and sugary beverages.

❖ Restrict Alcohol limit

Approximately more than 90% of the alcohol is metabolized in a liver. Liver enzymes metabolize alcohol into acetaldehyde which is a familiar cancer-causing chemical. Acknowledging acetaldehyde as a toxin, a liver converts it into a harmless substance known as acetate, which is later eliminated from a body.

Some studies have shown that consumption of alcohol from a low to moderate level is fruitful for heart health while its excessive drinking can cause many health problems like liver dysfunction that includes filtering waste and other toxins from a body.

Hence, limiting alcohol is one of the best ways to keep the body's detoxification system running strong. The recommended limit of alcohol from health authorities is to intake one drink per day for women and two drinks for men. But avoiding alcohol is the best solution.

❖ Concentrate on sleep

Each night a good quality sleep is very necessary to support the body's health and natural detoxification system. Sleep helps a brain to recharge itself and to remove toxic waste byproducts that have accumulated the whole day. One of the waste products is a protein known as beta-amyloid that takes part in the development of Alzheimer's disease.

Deprivation of sleep affects the functioning of a body. So, the body doesn't perform its role to remove toxins, so they start accumulating and affect different aspects of health. Short- and long-term health consequences regarding poor sleep involve stress, obesity, anxiety, type 2 diabetes, high blood pressure, and heart disease. One should sleep seven to nine hours per night daily to encourage good health. If a person finds difficulty in falling asleep and stays awake till late at night, then he should try to change his lifestyle like stick to a sleep schedule and limit blue light, don't use mobile and computers just before sleeping, etc. This will improve one's sleep. Hence, by taking adequate sleep, the body's brain will recharge, reorganize and eliminate toxins that accumulate throughout the day.

❖ **Use antioxidant-rich foods**

Antioxidants help in protecting body cells against damage caused by molecules known as free radicals. Oxidative stress is a condition that is caused by excessive production of free radicals. The body naturally produces these molecules for cellular processes like digestion but alcohol, tobacco, smoke, poor diet, and exposure to pollutants increase the production of free radicals in a body. This leads to different damages i.e. heart disease, liver disease, a certain type of cancer and asthma. Vitamin A, C and E, lutein, selenium, zeaxanthin, and lycopene are good antioxidants that are found in berries, fruits, nuts, spices, beverages, coca, and vegetables.

❖ **Consume food high in prebiotics**

The good health of a gut is very important for keeping body detoxification healthy. Intestinal cells contain a detoxification and excretion system that protects a gut and a body from harmful toxins such as chemicals. Good gut health initiated with prebiotics. This is a type of fibre that helps to feed good bacteria in a gut called probiotics. With the help of prebiotics, the good bacteria present in a body can produce nutrients known as short-chain fatty acids which are very favorable for health.

The ratio of good bacteria becomes unbalanced with bad bacteria if a person uses antibiotics, diet quality, and poor dental hygiene. This unhealthy shift in bacteria results in the weakening of the immune system and detoxification system leading to an increase in the risk of disease and inflammation. Good sources of prebiotics include tomatoes, oats, artichokes, garlic, bananas, onions, and asparagus.

❖ **Decrease the salt intake**

Excess use of salt can cause a body to retain excess fluid which will certainly affect the kidney and liver if a person doesn't drink enough water. Also, a body will start releasing an antidiuretic hormone that prevents a person from urinating. Increasing potassium intake will counterbalance the sodium effect. Potassium-rich foods include potatoes, spinach, squash, bananas and kidney beans.

- **Adopt an active lifestyle**

    Daily physical activity lowers inflammation and allows a body's detoxification system to work properly. A recommended duration of moderately intense exercise is 150 -300minutes a week i.e. brisk walking. If a person is doing an intense physical activity than 70-150min a week are enough i.e. running. This will reduce inflammation in the body and a body's detoxification system will improve leading to the proper functioning of a body and its strength to fight against diseases.

17.1 Detox with Caution

Despite enormous benefits and ease of detox processes that we can adapt, some cautions should be taken under consideration before going for any detox routine. Especially, in the case of thyroid conditions, unplanned and non-cautious detox can lead to more harm than good. People with thyroid dysfunction should practice any detox process after proper physician consultation and should keep a keen eye on their symptoms to prevent adverse reactions of detox on their body.

The reason behind this possible health damage of detox in thyroid dysfunction individual is the fact that the ability to detoxify toxins is largely dependent on the health of thyroid and liver. And due to thyroid hormonal imbalance, the health of the liver is compromised. Therefore, opting detoxification when the thyroid and liver are unhealthy is highly prohibited. As it can make the situation worse and can lead to irreversible damage to the liver and body and can lead to increase in hyperthyroidism and hypothyroidism. It is known that hypothyroidism blocks the essential detox pathways in the body and in such condition if you try to detox it will make things worse.

17.2 The Risk Associated with Detoxification with Hypothyroidism

There are two forms of toxins, water-soluble that can dissolve in water and fat-soluble that dissolute in only fats. Among the two, the water-soluble toxins are easy to remove and detoxify as they are removed from the body through perspiration and urine. While fat-soluble toxins cause various problems to the body as they are difficult to remove. And a special process, termed as the glucuronidation, is used by the body to get rid of fat-soluble toxins. This process of glucuronidation is carried out by the liver cells and efficiently removes fat-soluble toxins from the body by adding glucuronic acid to them. Once glucuronic acid is added to these toxins, they become water-soluble and are easily excreted.

This is the normal process of detoxification that takes place only in healthy individuals. People with Hashimotos's disease and hypothyroidism have a futile and nonfunctional glucuronidation process, which makes them unable to carry out the process of toxin detoxification.

As we already know that by taking a healthy diet and exercises only help to boost the already ongoing natural process of detoxification. So, if the process is hacked or halted, practising a detox regime can cause stress and dysfunction in the body. And hypothyroid patients who cannot eliminate the toxins can suffer from adverse effects if we attempt to force the toxins out of the fat cells. These toxins and harmful compounds end up dumped into the bloodstream and have deleterious effects on other organs of the body.

17.3 Thyroid-Friendly Ways to Boost Detoxification

It is advised that people with thyroid should be extra cautious before practicing detox protocols. Among the various available methods, one should select the protocol that heals the liver and thyroid and not become an added burden on the body. Thyroid individuals can significantly benefit from the detox process if they avoid the intake of toxins and take food that helps the liver in carrying out the detoxification process. There are certain key points that should be taken under special consideration by the patients of thyroid disorders that can help them do a healthy detox.

❖ Maintain the Thyroid Hormone (T3)

First and foremost, step in improving your health through detox is to regulate the level of thyroid hormone in the body. this is important because the liver is dependent on thyroid hormone (T3) to carry out various processes, including detoxification. The treatment of hypothyroidism by taking the T3 hormone can remove the inhibition of glucuronidation process that removes the toxins from the body and can lead to effective detox and improvement of general wellbeing.

❖ No to Polyunsaturated fatty acids PUFAs

A certain form of seed oil and polyunsaturated fats can lead to damage of the thyroid gland and compromises the detoxing ability of the liver. It is highly recommended that individuals with thyroid disorders should avoid PUFAs so that the detoxification process is not hindered.

❖ Yes to Carrot

Carrot is a must-have food for thyroid individuals. It is highly recommended that whatever diet or detox regime a thyroid patient is following, carrot salad or smoothie should be a part of it. Carrot helps in removing toxins from the liver and helps to improve symptoms of hypothyroidism.

❖ Eat your Proteins

Proteins are very nutritious and beneficial for thyroid individuals. It is recommended that one take a good amount (around 100 grams) of daily proteins that will help in improving thyroid and liver function and boost the process of detoxification. The best thyroid supportive protein sources include broth, collagen protein powder, and dairy.

❖ Drink Orange Juice

Orange juice is considered essential for liver function and the detox process. It is a must-have for thyroid patients as it helps the liver to efficiently produce glucuronic acid and remove harmful chemicals from the body. Orange juice improves the health of the thyroid gland and by combining it with other thyroid-boosting foods, it can exponentially boost the thyroid function.

18. Treatment for Thyroid Dysfunctions

Various therapeutic advancements have been made to manage thyroid dysfunction. These treatments primarily involve the use of drugs or hormones that increase or decrease the hormone-producing ability of the thyroid. As the two primary disorders of thyroid, hyperthyroidism and hypothyroidism, are caused by opposite reasons, the treatments of these conditions are also different. Some of the most widely used treatments of thyroid dysfunction are discussed in the next section.

18.1 Best Treatment Options for Hypothyroidism

As we know that hypothyroidism involves a deficiency of enough thyroid hormones. Hence, the treatment focuses on replacing this loss. There is no cure for hypothyroidism. Therefore, lifelong treatment is required to help a person feel better and decrease the risk of further related complications, such as heart disease.

One should very lucky once they and their doctors become able to figure out the best type and dosage of the medication for them. The most uncomfortable hypothyroidism symptoms include fatigue, weight gain and high cholesterol which can be reversed with proper treatment.

Some of the best hypothyroidism treatments options to be considered are discussed below:

18.1.1 Hormones replacement treatment

Mostly hypothyroidism is treated with thyroid hormone replacement therapy, and one of the most effective ways to treat hypothyroidism is with synthetic T4 medication. These hormones are almost the same as the natural T4 that is formed by the thyroid, but various factors can affect the exact dosage a person needs. This includes age, the severity of symptoms and a person's overall health profile.

Synthetic T4 is accessible in a prescription medication known as levothyroxine which is sold under brand names such as Levothroid and Synthroid. Many generic versions are also available. Switching the brands back and forth should be done carefully, as the doses may vary slightly.

Initially, when a person starts taking prescription

thyroxine hormones, a doctor prescribes a dosage based on the patient's blood test results. The higher the TSH and the lower the T4 levels then the larger will the required dosage. Dosage is set according to the weight of a person. Teenagers, children and the elder ones generally require smaller doses.

Setting the correct dosage is not a quick process. When a person starts taking medicine, a blood test between six and eight weeks are taken to observe if the hormone levels are normalizing. If the dosage doesn't adjust, the doctor will recheck the hormone level after another six to eight weeks. Once the thyroid hormone level stabilizes, a person will not be in a need of thyroid checkup for the next six months.

Synthetic thyroxine is taken daily in the morning on an empty stomach. One will have to wait 30 minutes before eating or drinking anything except that of water. If a person keeps on missing medicine doses, it will cause the thyroid to go unbalanced. But never take a double dose after skipping doses because this will raise the level of thyroid too much.

18.1.2 Medication with synthetic T3 and T4 hormones combination

Now a day such medicines are available that contain the combination of synthetic T4 and T3 hormones, but such medicines are often not recommended. Some patients feel an improvement in their health after using synthetic T4 alone because the thyroid can convert these hormones to T3 when required. However, the combination of synthetic T3 and T4 drugs causes anxiety. If a person is already suffering from any mental health disability, such side effects may even be more.

In some conditions, a doctor recommends an individual T3 medication known as Cytomel (liothyronine) in addition to levothyroxine.

18.2 The best treatment for hyperthyroidism

There are several existing treatments for hyperthyroidism. An appropriate approach depends on age, personal preference, physical condition, the severity of a disorder and the basic cause of hyperthyroidism. Feasible treatments include:

18.2.1 Beta-blockers

Usually, these drugs are used for the treatment of high blood pressure and don't affect the thyroid levels, but they help ease the symptoms of hyperthyroidism such as tremors, palpitations and rapid heart rate.

For the reason mentioned earlier, the doctor may advise a person to take these medicines to help the patient feel better until the thyroid levels become normal or near to normal. But this medication is usually not recommended for the people suffering from asthma. The side effects include fatigue and sexual dysfunction.

18.2.2 Surgery (Thyroidectomy)

This treatment is adopted in only a few cases as if a woman is pregnant or a person is unable to tolerate anti-thyroid medicines or does not want to go through a radioactive iodine therapy.

During thyroidectomy, a doctor removes most of a thyroid gland, but this surgery includes some risks i.e. damage to vocal cords and parathyroid glands. There are four small glands present on the back of a thyroid gland that helps a body to control the level of calcium in the blood may also get damage.

A person also will be needed a lifelong treatment with levothyroxine to provide a body the normal amount of thyroid hormone. If a parathyroid gland is also removed during surgery than a patient will also require medication to keep his blood calcium levels normal.

18.2.3 Radioactive iodine

In this treatment, radioactive iodine is taken by mouth, it gets absorbed by a thyroid gland, where it causes the gland to shrink. Usually, the symptoms abate within several months. The excess of radioactive iodine diminishes from the body in weeks to months.

Eventually, with the help of this treatment, the thyroid activity becomes slow enough to be considered underactive (hypothyroidism) and a patient may need to take medicine daily to replace thyroxine.

18.2.4 Anti-thyroid medications

During this treatment with medicines, the medication slowly starts reducing the symptoms of hyperthyroidism by preventing the thyroid gland from generating an excessive amount of hormones. This includes methimazole (Tapazole) and propylthiouracil. Usually, the symptoms begin to reduce within weeks to months but this treatment with anti-thyroid medications generally continues at least a year and often more than that.

There are some cases in which the problem clears up permanently but, in many cases, the people may experience a problem again. Both the medication drugs can cause serious liver damage and sometimes even leads to death. Because propylthiouracil has caused many cases of liver damage and one can only try to use this medicine when he is not able to tolerate methimazole.

Few cases also show that the people taking this medication who are allergic to these drugs may suffer from skin rashes, joint pains, hives or fever. These drugs may make a patient more susceptible to many infections.

REFERENCES

https://www.ncbi.nlm.nih.gov/books/NBK279388/

https://www.endocrineweb.com/conditions/thyroid-nodules/thyroid-gland-controls-bodys-metabolism-how-it-works-symptoms-hyperthyroid

https://www.endocrineweb.com/conditions/thyroid/how-your-thyroid-works

https://www.endocrineweb.com/conditions/thyroid/hypothyroidism-too-little-thyroid-hormone

https://www.mayoclinic.org/diseases-conditions/hashimotos-disease/symptoms-causes/syc-20351855

https://www.mayoclinic.org/diseases-conditions/hypothyroidism/symptoms-causes/syc-20350284

https://www.medicinenet.com/hyperthyroidism/article.htm

https://www.todaysdietitian.com/newarchives/070112p40.shtml

https://www.ncbi.nlm.nih.gov/pmc/articles/PMC3219766/

https://www.medicalnewstoday.com/articles/324819.php#foods-to-avoid-and-why

https://www.healthline.com/nutrition/hypothyroidism-diet#effects-on-metabolism

https://www.healthline.com/health/hyperthyroidism-diet#foods-to-avoid

https://www.healthline.com/health/hypothyroidism/diet-plan#3

https://www.sciencedirect.com/science/article/abs/pii/S0003426611000461

https://new.hindawi.com/journals/mi/2016/6757154/fig1/

https://www.health.harvard.edu/diseases-and-conditions/when-depression-starts-in-the-neck

https://www.ncbi.nlm.nih.gov/pmc/articles/PMC3246784/pdf/JTR2012-590648.pdf

https://www.cell.com/trends/endocrinology-metabolism/fulltext/S1043-2760(19)30107-9

https://www.ihcal.com/the-top-3-ways-to-flush-out-toxins-and-boost-thyroid-function/

http://www.amhsjournal.org/article.asp?issn=2321-4848;year=2015;volume=3;issue=2;spage=244;epage=246;aulast=Bansal

https://www.forefronthealth.com/thyroid-detox/

www.ingramcontent.com/pod-product-compliance
Lightning Source LLC
Chambersburg PA
CBHW052355220526
45465CB00003BA/1112